FAMILY NURSING: THE CASE OF CYSTIC FIBROSIS

Family Nursing:
The Case of Cystic Fibrosis

DOROTHY A. WHYTE
Department of Nursing Studies
University of Edinburgh

Avebury

Aldershot · Brookfield USA · Hong Kong · Singapore · Sydney

Published by
Avebury
Ashgate Publishing Limited
Gower House
Croft Road
Aldershot
Hants GU11 3HR
England

Ashgate Publishing Company
Old Post Road
Brookfield
Vermont 05036
USA

British Library Cataloguing in Publication Data

Whyte, Dorothy A.
    Family Nursing: The Case of Cystic Fibrosis
    I. Title
    610.7343

ISBN 1 85628 524 3

Printed and Bound in Great Britain by
Athenaeum Press Ltd, Newcastle upon Tyne.

Contents

Figures and tables

Foreword

It is a privilege and pleasure to write a brief foreword to this seminal contribution to nursing knowledge.

There cannot be many health professionals working in the community who do not intuitively recognise the significance of the family setting in relation to the care of individual patients or clients. This is particularly so in the case of long term chronic illness of a child. Yet this significance does not seem to have been appropriately addressed in nursing education, practice or management. Lack of credible knowledge may well be a major reason and this book makes a superb contribution to filling this gap.

The author attempted to answer the question 'What does it feel like to have a child with cystic fibrosis?' After all, how can the necessary support be offered without that knowledge? Through meticulous research using a complex mix of qualitative approaches she was able to penetrate deeply into the special problems, anxieties, fears, needs and hopes of families caring for a child with cystic fibrosis (CF), giving the child his or her own chance to speak. She gained insights which we cannot afford to ignore.

The research presented in this book emanated from the author's own nursing experience. It has the potential of underpinning future practice by giving substantive meaning to the concept of 'nursing support'. Moreover, the important newly created knowledge need not be confined to the support of families with CF children. Responsibly and validly, the author claims transferability of some pointers to any families with chronically ill children - not to be confused with generalisability of results.

The experience of chronic sorrow which must characterise all such families to some extent must be built into any careplan claiming to be helpful.

This book poses important challenges. It demonstrates the urgent need for knowledgeable doers of family nursing. I wished that it had been available when I was teaching and practising community nursing.

Lisbeth Hockey PhD, FRCN
Consultant Researcher, Edinburgh
November, 1993

Preface

This book is based on a PhD thesis, the work for which spanned the years between 1983 and 1989. Since that time there have been developments in many areas which impinge on this study. The temptation is to attempt a major re-write, particularly of the literature review, or else not to publish at all. I have decided to steer a middle course. The developments taking place suggest to me that an examination of nursing support for families caring for sick children in the community is in fact timely. Paediatric community nursing is gaining increasing professional recognition, (UKCC, 1993) and is of crucial importance in the Child Branch programmes of Project 2000 diploma courses. Work which contributes, albeit in a small way, to the knowledge base of an emerging discipline ought not to join the ranks of unpublished PhD theses.

I cannot ignore however the relevant works which have been published in the intervening years. Some of these have contributed to my ongoing thinking around this area of practice, teaching and research, and will hopefully be considered more fully in later writing.

Cystic fibrosis (CF) research is moving on in many areas, including the preliminary testing of gene therapy (Scott, 1993) and the provision of carrier detection screening programmes (Mennie et al, 1992). Awareness of psychosocial factors has increased, with the appointment by the Cystic Fibrosis Trust of Family Advice and Support Co-ordinators, and the organisation of a one-day conference in London in 1993 on psychosocial aspects of cystic fibrosis.

Theory and research related to psychological aspects of chronic illness has been most usefully reviewed by Christine Eiser (1990). By drawing extensively on published research and her own experience she has illuminated the whole area of coping, and helping families to cope, with the stresses imposed by chronic childhood disease. Another British text which makes a significant contribution is Neil Frude's Understanding Family Problems (1990). The chapter on the family unit gives a helpful explication of systems thinking applied to work with families, and the discussion of issues arising from childhood illness and handicap is highly relevant to nursing.

Bailey and Clarke (1989) and McHaffie (1992) have brought the coping literature into the nursing arena in the United Kingdom. These authors have synthesized knowledge on coping from various disciplines and theoretical stances, and applied it to nursing. Research in Finland on coping with cancer (Krause, 1991) and in Japan on coping behaviour of parents caring for children with cerebral palsy (Hiroise and Ueda, 1990) highlights the importance of this concept to understanding and supporting clients and demonstrates its transcultural applicability.

While the importance of including parents in the care of sick children continues to be stressed in nursing journals, there is still a gap in our knowledge of the effect of life-threatening illness on family functioning, and of how we as health professionals can assist families through their testing experience. Jennings (1992a) highlights the gaps between professional and client perspectives on the coping strategies used by mothers of children with tracheostomies, and by mothers of children with CF, caring for their children at home. Paediatric community nurses (PCN) were found to be the easiest of health professionals for mothers to talk to, but only one third of mothers had contact with a PCN. Jennings emphasises the need for specific training for paediatric community nursing, in agreement with the conclusions of this study, and discusses areas of support in which health professionals should become involved (Jennings, 1992b).

Much of the analysis of nursing work with families comes from North America. Yet many nurses and other health professionals have been developing expertise in this area in the United Kingdom. The field of family therapy has much to offer here, as some community psychiatric nurses have already recognised (MacPhail, 1988). A fascinating insight to the potential of integrating family therapy into in-patient paediatric settings is provided by John and Bradford (1991). Their commentary illustrates the point of my contention that paediatric nurses need a greater understanding of family functioning and systems thinking.

The feelings which initiated and drove this thesis are still with me. We need to understand more about how families cope with crises, and with the everyday burden of caring for a sick child. Crucially, those of us who have a professional responsibility to provide support, and/or teach others how they can develop family nursing skills, need to understand more about the kind of support which families find helpful. There is so much still to be discovered and shared. This book is offered, with only minor changes from the original thesis, as a small contribution to that body of knowledge.

My thanks are due to so many people who helped to make this work possible. First and foremost to the families from whose experience this study is derived. They shared their lives with me, and took an interest in the long gestation of the thesis.

Many professional colleagues gave support, showed interest and shared their thoughts. Most particularly, my academic supervisors - firstly Professor Annie Altschul, who asked many questions and helped me to focus my thinking. Her friendly interest continued to encourage me during her retirement. Professor Penny Prophit guided my approach to the research and helped me to develop my thoughts on nursing theory. Finally, Judith Brearley proved an exacting but immensely constructive critic and friend, whose expectations, suggestions and comments gave shape to the finished product.

In the practice arena, Muriel Balfour (nee Campbell) gave incalculable help by sharing her long experience, her reflections on that experience, and by providing support in the times when my own experience in practice proved emotionally difficult. Contact with colleagues through the Royal College of Nursing Society of Paediatric Nursing provided fresh insights and encouraged me to continue with the study.

Members of my family and friends helped in varying ways. In particular, I wish to thank my mother who gave patient practical support and my friend Pauline Baber for her painstaking proof-reading. My thanks also to Jennifer Clark and Linda Morris for their secretarial assistance in preparing this book for publication.

I wish also to acknowledge with thanks the financial assistance given by Edinburgh University Travel and Research Fund, and by the Gardner Bequest, which enabled me to attend the First International Family Nursing Conference in Calgary, Alberta, in 1988. This was not only an enjoyable experience but also proved influential in developing my thinking about families and nursing. Thanks also to the Moray Fund of Edinburgh University which provided the finance needed to prepare the work for publication.

Introduction

And a woman who held a babe against her
    bosom said,
Speak to us of children.
And he said
Your children are not your children.
They are the sons and daughters of life's
    longing for itself.
They come through you but not from you,
And though they are with you yet they
    belong not to you.
You may give them your love but not your
    thoughts,
For they have their own thoughts.
....
You are the bows from which your children
    as living arrows are sent forth.
The Archer sees the mark upon the path of
    the infinite, and He bends you with his
    might that His arrows may go swift and
    far.
So let your bending in the Archer's hand
    be for gladness;
For even as He loves the arrow that flies,
    so He loves also the bow that is
    stable.

(Gibran, *The Prophet*)

Chronic illness and handicap in childhood present painful paradoxes to our youth-orientated society. The normal process of growth and development towards independence and maturity is threatened, hindered or terminated. For families living with such a problem, stress is inevitable. Since children with chronic illness and handicap require health care services, nurses are involved in their care and are in a position to offer support. It is, however, an area of such complexity in terms of family interaction and coping with stress that nurses who do allow themselves to become involved over a period of time can become overwhelmed by the problems. Alternatively, they may find their nursing training inadequate to equip them to deal with situations requiring detailed psychological support (Robinson, 1988). The strategy of drawing in other professionals such as social workers or chaplains may provide a solution, but may be an example of the 'role-switching' described by Glaser and Strauss (1965, p.233) whereby nurses turn the family of terminally ill patients over to others to avoid disturbing scenes and to reduce involvement. It is evident that an ill child's welfare, even his survival, is dependent on an adequate level of family functioning. It seems important therefore that nurses, as first-line workers in providing care for the child and in teaching and supporting parents as the primary caregivers, understand the family dynamics involved in chronic childhood illness. From that understanding, a nursing response might be developed to help to strengthen families in their lengthy, intensely demanding commitment to the care of a chronically ill member. Kodakek's (1979) comment is pertinent:

> There is a direct role for the nurse in treating the child, but there is an equally important supportive role for the nurse with the family. (p.367)

Background to the study

The seeds of the concern which led to this study were sown some years ago when I was a health visitor student in Glasgow. Because of my paediatric nursing background I was asked to visit a family in which there was a child with cystic fibrosis. I found an intensely sad situation in which an older brother had already died of cystic fibrosis and the 12-year old patient, a 'respiratory cripple', had a resigned air of waiting for his turn to come. His mother seemed to share the sense of hopelessness. The lack of nursing support up to that time struck me forcibly. Possible reasons for this may have been a sense of inadequacy in such a dire situation, a lack of knowledge about a disease which at that time was mainly confined to chilhood, or anxiety about personal involvement. I was perplexed and grieved by many aspects of the situation, but my involvement was limited by its essentially short-term nature.

When the opportunity arose, in the context of an honorary appointment with the local Health Board, to carry a small caseload of children with cystic fibrosis, I resolved to study the nursing situation closely. From the beginning, therefore, I kept detailed notes of home visits and contacts in hospital or clinic. The problem area was large and complex.

Cystic fibrosis (CF) is a permanent, non-curable condition; the commonest serious inherited disorder in Caucasian races. The genetic defect is as yet non-reversible. The long-awaited break-through in research came in September 1989 with the precise location of the gene. While this offers progress in detection of the carrier state, and earlier and more accurate diagnosis, the benefits for those who have the disease may not be realised for some years to come. The digestive problems and lung infections currently require constant, vigorous therapy. This in itself places a considerable burden on a family's coping mechanisms, but the factor which makes the burden almost intolerable is the knowledge that the condition is life-threatening. Most commonly, the diagnosis follows investigation of persistent respiratory infection and failure to thrive, typically a hungry child who has frequenty bulky stools. Treatment cannot offer a cure, but early diagnosis and the institution of vigorous therapy has resulted in increased life expectancy. The essential characteristics, then, are of a pathological condition which can be treated but not cured, which is long-term but with a varying course, which requires intensive daily therapy in order to maintain a reasonable quality as well as quantity of life - and which is ultimately life-threatening.

The implications for the family of caring for a child with CF has been the subject of a good deal of research. As I worked with the families and explored the literature on cystic fibrosis I became convinced that there remained a need for clearer insights to the family experience than were already available. Since the focus of my concern was the nursing contribution to support of the family through the experience of caring for their child, it seemed important to make a detailed longitudinal study of the effect of the child's illness on family interaction and of the interaction between nurse and family.

The study began in 1983 and for three years full and accurate field notes of all interactions with the families were kept. During this time I was searching for the most appropriate way to organise the research approach, and reviewing literature directly related to CF and, more generally, to the area of chronic illness in childhood. This, in turn, led to literature on families and some of the concepts such as crisis, coping and loss which, it was becoming clear, were important.

The research base for the nursing care of children with chonic conditions is far from strong (Muller et al, 1986; Hirschfeld and Krulik, 1985; Sinclair and Whyte, 1987). There is a considerable literature, however, by workers from other health care disciplines on families who have a child with cystic fibrosis, particularly the work of Burton (1975), Bywater (1981), and McCollum and Gibson (1970).

While Stein and Jessop (1982) argued that the commonalities of the different chronic illnesses outweigh the difference according to diagnosis in regard to caregiving, Tizard (1978) contended that in order to further research to improve practice social scientists must learn to concentrate on highly specific problems (p.132). He commented that medical scientists long ago abandoned attempts to put the whole world to rights. Nurses, too, are increasingly finding themselves drawn into specialist roles and it makes sense, therefore, to use cystic fibrosis as a paradigm, with the possibility of later being able to apply some of the findings to other chronic illnesses.

The word 'chronic' has within it the concept of time and the Oxford Dictionary defines it as lingering or lasting a long time. Time has a particular significance in the lives of those coping with life-threatening disease such as cystic fibrosis. Mattsson's (1972) definition is helpful and can be readily applied to CF:

> Chronic illness refers to a disorder with a protracted course which can be progressive and fatal or associated with a relatively normal life span despite impaired physical and mental functioning. Such a disease frequently shows periods of acute exacerbations requiring intensive medical attention. (p.801)

In looking at the psychosocial implications of CF, the work of McCollum and Gibson (1970) was particularly useful for its introduction of the stages of adaptation through which families progress when they are dealing with CF. The review led on to a consideration of the literature on the family, and two particularly useful texts here were those of Will and Wrate (1985) and Minuchin (1974), with their work on family structure and ways of dealing with developmental tasks. Consideration of vulnerable families and hazardous events led to a review of the literature on crisis, which led in turn to study of coping and of the concept of transitions in family life. The final area to be studied was loss, death and bereavement, with an attempt to limit the focus to the death of a child and anticipatory grieving. All of these conceptual areas have a considerable literature and it was necessary to restrict the review to key texts in the general area and to home in on the issues related to childhood illness, and, where possible, to CF in particular. Reflection on the literature and on my experience with the families led gradually to the formulation of the research questions.

The research questions

My involvement with the families was firstly as a nurse with expert knowledge in the area of CF and with a concern for the welfare of the whole family. The parents knew from the initial visit that I had a research interest in CF and how it affected family life. I entered the field with few preconceived ideas, but gradually research questions emerged and my contact with families became more purposeful, particularly with regard to the questions asked and the exploration of feelings and perceptions.

1   How do family members respond to the genetic implications of cystic fibrosis (CF)?

2   How do families respond to the life-threatening nature of CF?

3   How does time affect the way families perceive and experience the illness?

4   How do family members find meaning in their experience of CF?

5   What events precipitate crises and what constitutes the chronic burden of care in the lives of families caring for a child with CF?

6   How does caring for a child with CF affect interaction and the coping response of families?

7   What is the impact of CF on individual family members and on their coping response?

8   What support networks do families use in relation to caring for the child with CF?

9   What support would families caring for a child with CF like to have?

The research approach

The research strategy appropriate to such an exploration was an ethnographic and phenomenological approach with its commitment to studying the subjects' views of their experience. Hammersley and Atkinson's (1983) very useful exposition of the principles of ethnography was particularly influential in guiding the research strategy. The work of Glaser and Strauss (1967) with their development of grounded theory shed light on the difficult business of data analysis. Case study research involves intensive observation of an individual or a group and thus provided an appropriate framework for the research. Meier and Pugh (1986) reviewed the application of the case study method in other practice-based disciplines and concluded that this method presented "... a viable research strategy for investigation of client-centred clinical phenomena within the domain of nursing" (p.200). This approach allowed for the collection of data from a variety of sources, which was in keeping with the strategy which had been adopted. Elements of life history interviewing using a tape recorder were used towards the end of the study period with the aim of increasing the breadth and depth of the data.

Presentation of data

The results of the first stage of data analysis takes the form of family profiles in which the four families are introduced and their progress through the stages of adaptation related to CF is narrated. Much of this chapter contains direct quotations from the life history interviews, allowing the family members to tell their own stories. There is also an assessment of the way in which the families have dealt with basic and developmental tasks, and with the crises which they experienced.

There follows a further analysis of the data in which the research questions are considered through an examination of the experience of the subject families. Using a grounded theory approach, concepts are generated and theoretical perspectives developed. This leads in to the final discussion of nursing theory and the implications of the study for nursing practice, management and education. Areas for further research are considered.

The justification for this study lay in the perception which I gained, and which was borne out by the literature search, that families bearing the burden of care of a child with a chronic life-threatening illness such as cystic fibrosis required support. Nurses were likely to be involved with such families and, in view of the complexity of the nursing situation, it seemed important to develop understanding of the families' experience. Such an understanding might provide a theoretical base from which the concept of nursing support could be clarified.

Chapter one:
Literature review

In this chapter the definition of chronic illness is explored and related to the specific nature of cystic fibrosis. The aetiology, pathology, clinical features and treatment of cystic fibrosis are briefly described. The psychosocial problems related to this condition are examined in the light of research studies. In view of its centrality to the questions raised by this study, there follows a consideration of the family and the general systems approach to family functioning. The concepts of crisis and coping are analysed in general terms and related to studies of families coping with cystic fibrosis. Finally, the concepts of loss and bereavement are studied, focusing primarily on the anticipated loss of a child and the particular case of cystic fibrosis as a cause of psychosocial transition for the family. It will be appreciated that there is a vast literature in each of these subject areas and I have attempted in each case to give a general view of the topic then to focus more closely on the immediate concern, that is, the child and the family coping with cystic fibrosis (CF). The main sources are research papers but research-based textbooks, news sheets, educational booklets and autobiographies have also been used where they furnished useful information or insight. Because of the rapid progress of research it has been necessary to update some of the information found in the original literature search.

Chronic illness in childhood

Several writers have drawn attention to the changing patterns of health care whereby improved social conditions, immunisation, and advanced therapeutic regimes and technology have reduced infant and child mortality rates but increased the proportion of children requiring long-term care (Stein and Jessop, 1982; Hirschfeld and Krulik, 1985; Younghusband et al, 1970; Wright and Leahey, 1987).

Chronic illness has been defined as:

All impairments and deviations from normal which have one or more of the following characteristics: are permanent; leave residual disability; are caused by non-reversible pathological alterations; may require special training ay be expected to require a long period of supervision, observation or care.

(National Commission on Chronic Illness, 1956)

This is a very broad definition which could include a wide range of disorders in childhood. It is, however, so wide as to be not altogether helpful. The individual with spina bifida would usually have all the characteristics of chronic illness by the above definition, though parents may well prefer to think of their child as having a disability or a handicap rather than a chronic illness; and, indeed, such a preference would be supported by clinical observation. Individuals who have had surgery for spina bifida may have limitations, may have to deal with intercurrent infections and may have no prospect of a 'normal' lifestyle, but they would not regard themselves as being 'chronically ill'. The term carries connotations of invalidity, frailty, recurring illness and increasing disability. The picture portrayed is not at all that of a child with a disability such as diabetes mellitus, where the emphasis is on education for healthy independence, yet this condition would also have the characteristics of the definition.

Mattsson's (1972) definition referred to in the Introduction is more helpful:

Chronic illness refers to a disorder with a protracted course which can be progressive and fatal or associated with a relatively normal life span despite impaired physical and mental functioning. Such a disease frequently shows periods of acute exacerbations requiring intensive medical attention."
(p.801)

This definition again indicates something of the variations in the course and severity of chronic illness, but is more useful than the first definition given which could include minor physical defects such as a squint or the loss of a finger. Neill (1979) emphasised that chronic physical illness does not always presume a handicap. The extent of handicap relates to the obstacles to fulfilment of the child's potential imposed by the disability itself and by the changes in the environment brought about by the disability (p.445). This perspective on handicap is useful in the consideration of the effects on the child of having cystic fibrosis and the additional influences on the child caused by the effect of the illness on his family and social environment.

Craig and Edwards (1983) in their elegant development of an eclectic model

8

for nursing patients with chronic illness stated:

> The trajectory of chronic illness is in a generally downwards direction, although the rate of progression of the trajectory may vary as plateaux and remissions occur. The individual and his family move through the process of continual adjustment to changes in the course of the disease towards a goal of adaptation. (p.397)

Their definition of adaptation (after Feldman) is as follows:

> Coming to terms with the reality of chronic illness as a state of being, discarding false hope and destructive hopelessness and restructuring the environment in which one now functions. Adaptation implies the reorganization and acceptance of self so that there is a meaning and purpose to living that transcends the limitations imposed by the illness. (p.399)

Roy (1983), applying her adaptation theory of nursing to family health, gave the following definition:

> Adaptation ... is the individual's response to the environment that promote the person's general goals, including survival, growth, reproduction, and mastery, or, more simply, it is behaviour that maintains the integrity of the individual. (p.268)

She saw adaptation as freeing energy from inadequate or inappropriate coping attempts, thereby promoting health. This freedom to restructure and re-organise, incorporating the child's illness and treatment as part of the reality of family life, is the meaning of the term 'adaptation' as it is used in this study.

In a study of social work and chronic illness, Hardiker and Tod (1982) made the distinction between illness and disease. Disease was said to refer to the presence of pathological abnormality and to be indicated by signs such as swelling, irregular temperature or abnormal blood counts. Illness was more related to the individual's feeling of discomfort and recourse to medical treatment (p.642). This distinction linked illness with the concept of the sick role. Features of chronic illness highlighted in this paper were its invisibility and uncertainty. Issues of self-esteem and stigma were also identified. Living with uncertainty and weariness was said to sum up the burden of chronic illness (p.647). Cystic fibrosis has all the features of chronic illness and, in this chapter, it is examined both as a disease, in terms of its pathological features, and as in illness, in terms of its effect on the life of the child and his family.

9

Cystic fibrosis

Cystic fibrosis is a permanent, non-curable condition. It is estimated that around 400 new CF cases are diagnosed each year in the United Kingdom and in 1984 there were an estimated 6,000 sufferers (Capewell, 1986, OHE, p.10). The genetic defect is as yet non-reversible and the resultant lung infections do eventually leave disability. The child and his parents require special training in physiotherapy techniques to improve lung function and reduce the susceptibility to infection. Special care is essential throughout life. The condition therefore shows all the characteristics of chronic illness as defined by the National Commission. An additional important aspect referred to in Mattsson's definition is that it is life-threatening. This is a major factor when considering the impact on the family. It is this aspect which causes emotional pain out of all proportion to the degree of disability caused initially by the illness. It is in most instances a long-term condition. With early diagnosis and vigorous therapy many individuals with cystic fibrosis reach adult life. Landau (1987) found that more than 50% of people with CF currently lived until they were at least 20. In its advanced stages it does meet the picture of frailty and disablement suggested by the term 'chronic illness', but in the earlier years there may be the appearance of a healthy, active youngster.

Aetiology

Cystic fibrosis was first clearly described in the 1930's by Fanconi, working in Switzerland, and Anderson in Baltimore (Harris and Super, 1987, p.10). It is the commonest serious inherited disorder affecting the Caucasian population. The incidence in races other than Caucasian is unknown but it has been diagnosed in Indians, Japanese, Negroes and Arabs (McCrae, 1984, p.511). In view of the diagnostic difficulty, it seems possible that the incidence in other races may be higher than was previously believed. The pattern of inheritance is autosomal recessive, which means that both parents must be carriers of the defective gene, though their own health is unaffected. It is estimated that, in the Caucasian population, 1 in 20 individuals carry the deleterious gene and that approximately 1 in 400 marriages are at risk of producing an affected child. The pattern of inheritance is illustrated in Figure 1; in every pregnancy there is a 1:4 chance of a child having CF. McCrae (1984) made the point that with the recognition of CF in races other than Caucasian and the longer survival rates in areas where there are good paediatric services, the total clinical 'burden' of CF is increasing markedly (p.512).

Now that the basic protein defect has been identified the diagnosis of CF can be more accurate and better screening tests for carriers can be devised. The promise of better treatments and even gene therapy for individuals who have the disease offers real encouragement to families, although it is likely to be some years before such developments become reality (Science, 1989, p.923). Raeburn (1983) emphasised the importance of sensitive genetic counselling for parents, pointing out that a normal response to unwelcome news may seriously interfere with the parents' ability to communicate which, if not recognised and accepted, may damage their ongoing relationship with health professionals (p.7).

Pathology

The manifestations of the disease are diverse and include abnormality of all the exocrine glands, but the principal effects are seen in the lungs and respiratory tract, the digestive system and the sweat. For many years, the thick, sticky mucus was regarded as pathognomic of CF, hence the term 'mucoviscidosis', but research has failed to produce consistent evidence of abnormality of the mucus itself. It seems likely that the abnormalities described were secondary to the presence of lung infection (Harris and Super, 1987, p.96). It is the susceptibility to respiratory infections which becomes debilitating and life-threatening, and which is associated with late cardiovascular complications.

The respiratory infection begins in the peripheral airways but extends to larger airways and progresses to bronchiectasis, where bronchi are dilated, with associated infection and lobular collapse. Common pathogens in the early stages are staphylococcus aureus and haemophilus influenzae. The most difficult micro-organism to eradicate is pseudomonas aeruginosa and more recently, pseudomonas cepacia; these cause persistent infection in the later stages of the disease (Batten and Matthew, 1983, p.106), (Gladman et al, 1992). Respiratory complications which may be seen as the disease progresses include cor pulmonale, haemoptysis, emphysema and pneumothorax. Pulmonary function tests assist in the monitoring of the child's respiratory status. Bronchial hyperreactivity is common in patients with CF, probably related to the continuous inflammation and infection of the bronchial tree and noted to occur more frequently in patients with poor pulmonary function (Levison et al, 1983, p.65).

In the digestive system the pancreatic cells are replaced with fibrous scar tissue and production of pancreatic enzymes decreases. There is a failure of production of water and bicarbonate so that the pH of the duodenal contents is inadequately changed from the acidic pH of stomach contents to the alkaline pH at which pancreatic enzymes function best (Harris and Super, 1987, p.25). The resultant deficiency of enzymes causes a form of malabsorption. Cirrhosis of the liver occurs in about 5% of people with CF (Harris and Super, 1987, p.30). The fibrous tissue laid down can damage liver cells and cause portal hypertension. In the neonatal period inspissated meconium can cause intestinal obstruction in the

11

distal ileum which may be complicated by volvulus or perforation. The term 'meconium ileus equivalent' is used to describe a syndrome of small-intestinal obstruction unique to CF which can cause acute or chronic bowel obstruction later in life.

Immunological abnormalities have been found in association with CF and it is likely that they contribute to tissue damage and increasing severity of the disease. A mild degree of diabetes mellitus is a later development experienced by some individuals with CF. Lebenthal and Baswell (1983, p.303) recorded 1-2% in the paediatric population increasing to 13% of patients over 25 years of age, with larger numbers showing impaired glucose tolerance. It is presumed to result from increasing damage to the islet cells as the pancreatic lesion progresses.

There is a sweating abnormality which has proved helpful for the development of diagnostic techniques. The sweat has a raised level of chloride and sodium electrolytes, over 70 and 60 mmol/1 respectively, thought to be due to an unknown inhibiting factor reducing re-absorption of these electrolytes by the duct cells. The sweat test was considered the single most reliable procedure in the diagnosis of CF, until genetic mapping became available, although there is potential for error and most centres require at least two positive results. The principle of the test is the use of iontophoresis to enhance the penetration of the skin by pilocarpine, which stimulates the sweat glands (Kuzemko and Heeley, 1983, p.16)

Reproduction is affected in that over 90% of males with CF are sterile. There is a failure in development of the epididymis, seminal vesicles and vas deferens resulting in absence of sperm. The testes themselves develop normally and produce male sex hormones, leading to normal sexual development, drive and performance (Walters and Hodson, 1987, p.6). Fertility in the female may be slightly reduced due to viscid cervical mucus forming a barrier to the passage of sperm, or due to low body weight, but for practical purposes the woman with CF can expect to be fully fertile, accepting that other causes of infertility unrelated to CF could affect her as much as anyone in the general population.

Clinical features

The diagnosis may be made following presentation of meconium ileus in the neonatal period or rectal prolapse in an infant or young child. Alternatively, follow-up of siblings of affected children can provide a diagnosis in an apparently healthy child. Most commonly, however, the diagnosis follows investigation of persistent respiratory infection and failure to thrive. In some cases the respiratory infections are not a dominant feature and the child presents for investigation of frequent, fatty, foul-smelling stools, abdominal distension and failure to thrive. Because of the high sodium concentration in the sweat, parents may notice that their child tastes salty when kissed. Textbooks often refer to the voracious appetite of the CF child, which may be a feature before diagnosis, but after treatment starts parents more often complain of the child being anorexic.

Treatment and outcome

Treatment cannot offer a cure, but early diagnosis and institution of vigorous therapy has dramatically changed the course of the illness. Shwachman et al (1970) reported a 20-year study which illustrated this change. Prior to 1939 more than 85% of patients were dead by the end of the second year of life. By 1969, the mean age of death was 15 years; of the total of 130 cases in the study commenced in 1949, 29 had died. Social factors were reckoned to have contributed to four of these deaths.

Stern et al (1976), following the course of 95 patients in Cleveland, Ohio, reported a similar improvement in life expectancy and attempted also to assess morbidity, academic success, social adaptation and vocational achievement. At the end of the 17-year study, 28 of the 95 patients had died, the range of age at death being 6-24 years. All of the post-mortem findings showed typical pulmonary and pancreatic changes, and 18 of the 21 examinations showed right ventricular hypertrophy. Other major findings included duodenal ulcer and cirrhosis. Of the survivors, 33 had reached 18 years of age. Only one patient was reported as disabled. Seven patients had married; no pregnancies had occurred. Work and school attendance had been good among the young adults.

In the discussion of these findings, the researchers questioned the assumption that improved antimicrobial therapy was the most important, if not the only, factor in the improved prognosis. Thirty-three per cent of their patient population had received no, or only one, course of the newer antibiotics. Early institution of aggressive therapy before substantial pulmonary disease became established, conscientious follow-up by knowledgeable physicians, 24-hour access to specialised care and optimal inpatient facilities were felt to be the major factors in the control of CF. There was clearly a very committed hospital-based team where the physician's role was central; psychological problems were reportedly discussed openly and consultation obtained if indicated. Adults continued to be cared for by paediatricians and all patients had 24-hour access to a centre physician. Early hospital admission for treatment of pulmonary infection was encouraged and some patients continued to work full-time during a period of hospitalisation.

Stern et al's study sets the scene of the modern therapeutic approach to cystic fibrosis but also raises questions about such issues as transition to adult services and home care. New therapies continue to be developed. The newer preparations of enteric-coated pancreatin allow the use of lower total dosages. Greater

13

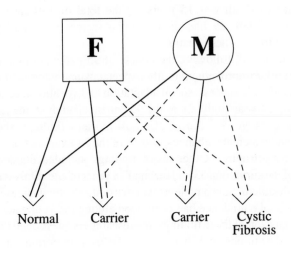

Figure 1
*Manner of inheritance in cystic fibrosis adapted from Office Health
Economics (1986) Cystic fibrosis p.10*

understanding of calorie requirements has influenced a policy of few dietary restrictions. Intravenous lines with an implantable device such as 'Portacath' have enhanced the efficacy and convenience of antibiotic therapy and facilitated home treatment. The Forced Expiratory Technique offers independence in the management of physiotherapy, allowing greater freedom to CF sufferers. Heart-lung transplants have been achieved. Nevertheless, cystic fibrosis continues to pose an ongoing and major threat to health and life. It is clear, too, that the economic burden is increasing as technology advances, whether the cost is borne by the family or by the State. In the following section the implications for child and family of such a diagnosis will be considered.

Psychosocial effects of cystic fibrosis

The earliest reported study of the psychosocial aspects of this disease appeared in the journal *Pediatrics* (Turk, 1964). The study was undertaken to determine whether or not families of children with CF experienced difficulties in meeting family needs and in maintaining family relationships. A self-administered questionnaire was issued to 28 parents of 25 families, that is, three fathers as well as 25 mothers participated. The questions were partly closed and partly open-ended, and attempted to identify specific areas of social and emotional deprivation, and problems in communication between family members. The findings indicated that parents felt deprived of time and energy to engage in leisure activities for the family, time to be alone with spouse, time for self, and time and energy to engage in adult activities. Significant difficulties in communication existed in these families, to the extent that Turk coined the oft-quoted phrase 'web of silence' in which each member of the family was locked in to his own frustrations, unable to discuss the demands posed by CF. Finances, prognosis and diet were said to head the list of subjects difficult to discuss. (This was in spite of the fact that this group did not have to meet hospital or medication expenses). The writer acknowledged that there had to date been no attempt to study the problems of families including children with other life-threatening diseases, nor was there any reference to comparable communication problems or frustrations in family relationships where the problem of chronic illness did not exist.

Stages of adaptation to chronic illness

Researchers following Turk's study looked at the increasing lifespan of CF children and suggested that there was a danger that this could constitute little more than an attenuated death, with a highly destructive impact upon the family (McCollum and Gibson, 1970). Their study investigated 56 families with 65 children with CF and obtained information from multiple-choice questionnaires, from in-depth interviews and from group discussions with parents. McCollum and Gibson identified four stages of adaptation through which parents progressed: pre-diagnostic; confrontational; long-term adaptive; and terminal. The terminal stage was not dealt with in the paper as none in the group had reached that point, but the other stages gave valuable insight to the stresses experienced by parents. As they later proved useful in the organisation of data in the case studies, they are described in some detail here.

The pre-diagnostic stage was characterised by anxiety about symptoms, misdiagnoses, a lack of improvement and a growing distrust of, and hostility towards, the medical profession. The problems of feeding disturbance, being difficult to comfort, fussiness and failing to thrive had a detrimental effect on the mother-infant relationship. Mothers expressed feelings of self-doubt at their failure to nurture the infant successfully, leading to feelings of despair and hostility towards the infant. These feelings were reinforced by the foul stools and the persistent cough.

The confrontational stage followed confirmation of the diagnosis and was a period of acute stress. The threat of a potentially fatal illness in their child led parents into an acute anticipatory mourning reaction. As well as the central issue of the possible loss of their child, there arose the questions of adding to their family and of the possibility that other members of the family might also be afflicted. Other focal points for stress were finance (McCollum and Gibson estimated a possible cost of $10,000 per child per annum for treatment of CF), and housing which had to be within reach of a medical centre and therapeutic techniques. It is worth noting that the mist tent was identified as a particular source of stress; not only did it necessitate a separate room which then suffered the effects of a constantly damp environment, but parents also reported fantasies that the child would suffocate, that it was "isolating, damp and chilly" and that the reduction of visual contact was frightening (p.575). This aspect of home treatment was never incorporated in the home care programme of some centres in the United Kingdom and the use of intermittent nebulisers is now widely favoured.

The long-term adaptive phase was described as one in which there was a fluctuating balance between intercurrent mourning and denial of prognosis. Denial as a useful defence was invariably impeded by obstructive characteristics of the disease such as the smell of stools and flatus which was perceived as permeating the household, the cough, time spent on therapy and sleep disturbance. The danger of respiratory infections was a chronic focus of apprehension. For the children, it was harder to gain independence and as they developed they became more sensitive to their 'differentness' and showed an emerging awareness of their prognosis. The 'web of silence' was evident again in that 28% of the children asked no questions of their parents about the illness and approximately a third of the parents admitted that they avoided providing information for the child for fear of direct questions about death which they felt unable to face. It was noted that information gained from the media, or in relation to fund-raising, and comments made by school-mates or siblings could cause distress to the children. It was observed with concern that, in adolescence, school avoidance was permitted by parents if not encouraged and compliance with therapy was less, seeming to indicate underlying feelings of hopelessness.

The writers concluded that group meetings of parents with the paediatrician and social worker allowed a sharing of information , anxieties and solutions, although only limited exposure of fears was appropriate within such a group. Deeper issues could be explored in individual interviews and the point was made that such interaction helped professionals to deepen their own insights into the problems of families they were trying to help (p.578).

These early studies have been criticised for their lack of objective measurement and small samples, but they provided rich insight to the experience of families coping with CF. They also identified key issues which helped to clarify the research questions. McCollum and Gibson's study provided an organising famework for handling the data from the family studies.

Other studies which offered similar frameworks were those by Harrisson (1977) and Rolland (1988). Harrisson used an approach modified from a major disaster framework to describe the sequence of personal adjustments to the impact of illness. These were: warning or threat; impact; inventory or adjustment; and terminal, closely reflecting McCollum and Gibson's four stages. A further illuminating description of the stages of chronic illness was found in the time phases suggested by Rolland (1984, p.30). He argued that each phase had its own psychosocial tasks which required different strengths and attitudes of the family concerned. The psychosocial themes in the natural history of chronic disease consisted of three phases: crisis, chronic, and terminal. The crisis phase was sub-divided into a pre-diagnostic stage and an initial adjustment period, the chronic phase was termed the 'long haul' and the terminal phase included the pre-terminal stage, death, mourning and resolution of loss. It can be seen from Figure 2 that Rolland's first two stages contained the elements of McCollum and Gibson's first three stages. Rolland's expansion of the terminal stage was helpful; McCollum and Gibson's study did not include children in this stage and, in my study, only one child might be considered to be in a pre-terminal stage. The congruence of these approaches, spanning a number of years and derived from different perspectives, validates the concept of stages of adaptation as a theme of the natural history of chronic illness.

Effect of cystic fibrosis on family interaction and functioning:
Parents and affected child.

Parallel studies in Northern Ireland and Scotland in the 1970's looked at the experience of families caring for a child with cystic fibrosis (Burton, 1975; Cull, 1974). Burton reviewed the early North American studies which reported severe stress in CF families, resulting in depression, anxiety and marital tension, but criticised them on the basis that they had attributed all family difficulties to the fact that a child had cystic fibrosis, where pre-existing conditions or general financial stresses may have had just as severe an impact on family functioning.

Burton's study had two aims: firstly, to assess the problems posed by CF for families living in a welfare state where one would not expect an additional financial burden; and, secondly, to study the ways in which parents and children were able to surmount the anxieties and stresses they underwent. Fifty-three families with one or more children with CF participated. These formed the total population of CF families in Northern Ireland and represented widely differing economic and social circumstances. The Scottish study had a similar sample size and social class range. (A criticism of some of the American studies is the unrepresentative nature of their sample). Both studies involved interviews with family members and the use of objective tests such as Taylor's Manifest Anxiety Scale and the Children's Manifest Anxiety Scale. Cull (p.124) herself questioned the validity of these tests, in that the first assessed anxiety-proneness rather than anxiety levels related to a specific anxiety-producing situation while the second relied on acquiescent response in children who may well have wanted to please the interviewer. Both studies also used control groups. In Burton's study, the severely handicapped subject children were matched with children equally handicapped by other disorders such as asthma or heart conditions. Cull matched her subject group with families who were caring for a child with coeliac disease.

Interviews in both studies were conducted in the home and on average each family was visited four times; fathers were normally interviewed on one of these occasions. Interview schedules were devised, the emphasis being on the parents' methods of overcoming the difficulties they faced. The reactions of younger children were studied by asking the mother to complete a Vineland Social Maturity Scale. Older children were interviewed in their own home and asked to complete a variety of tests related to scholastic ability and level of anxiety. Class teachers were also asked to use a Bristol Social Adjustment Guide and the

McCollum and Gibson (1970)	Harrison (1977)	Rolland (1988)
Pre-diagnostic	Warning or Threat	Pre-diagnostic
Confrontational	Impact	Initial Crisis Adjustment
Long-term Adaptive	Inventory or Adjustment	Chronic "the long haul"
Terminal	Terminal	Pre-terminal Death Terminal Mourning Resolution of loss

Figure 2

Stages of adaption to chronic illness: comparative approaches

results were compared with those of children matched with the subject children in terms of intellectual potential, academic attainment, sex, age, socio-economic status, ordinal position in the family and school attendance.

Communication

The interviews yielded a wealth of information and, in both studies, family communication was seen to be deleteriously affected. Burton (p.129) reported 16% of mothers and 25% of fathers feeling unable to fully talk over the illness with one another. Thirty per cent of women and 65% of men were unable to discuss it fully with family members and with increasing social distance communication diminished further, for example, 91% of men felt unable to communication fully with their general practitioner about the illness. The reluctance to communicate with their partner was often explained in terms of wishing to spare the other further worry. Reticence between parents and child was clearly related to the threatening aspects of the disease. One mother was quoted as saying, "I feel I could harm her by saying the wrong things" (p.137).

Burton identified several factors which militated against good parent-child communication. These were related to guilt on the mother's part, on the father's part to a sense that the marriage was not strengthened by experience of the disease, and to the loss of a previous child. These factors caused an emotional discomfort which adversely affected the parent's ability to communicate with the child and, not surprisingly, this was reflected in the child's level of communication concerning his illness. It was felt that parents needed help in knowing how to give age-appropriate and anxiety-allaying explanations to their children (p.137).

Cull (1984, p.595) also noted that family communication was inhibited and that this appeared to have a deleterious effect on the mother's health and on the marital relationship. She recognised, however, that her findings on communication in families had to be viewed with caution since personality factors, rather than the presence of childhood illness, were shown to be the main determinants of the fathers' ability to communicate with their wives.

Social factors

The financial burden of caring for a child with CF in a welfare state was difficult to estimate and some families felt that there was no additional expense, but others could estimate additional sums in relation to travel for clinic appointments, better foodstuffs and loss of earnings. In many cases the burden did not seem excessive, but in families where the financial budget was already exceedingly tight, the additional strains of caring for the ill child had a severely detrimental effect on family relationships and on the care experienced by the child. In relation to work difficulties, few mothers in Northern Ireland felt that their domestic work, or their work outside the home, was seriously affected by the necessity of caring for the sick child. Twenty-seven per cent of fathers, however, had to give up work at some time to help in caring for the sick child or the other children. While this was not resented, it was seen to create some work difficulties. In the Scottish study, 13 parents - 12 fathers and one mother - had lost work for reasons directly related to CF. It was concluded that there were some financial pressures resulting from caring for the sick child. Reasons related to CF were given to account for the fact that 20% of families had not been able to take holidays (Cull, 1974, p.225).

In terms of general hardship, mothers reported loss of energy, less spare time and less fun in life, with less time to spend with their spouse and less spending money, but these hardships were generally accepted philosophically and parents commented on the benefit of the National Health Service.

The affected child

In the ongoing stage of coping with the illness, Burton found the following problems related to pre-school age children: behaviour problems, that is, excessive temper tantrums; feeding problems; toileting problems, particularly associated with foul-smelling stools; sleep disorders; and rectal prolapse, the latter causing much distress to parents and child. A considerable dislike of physiotherapy was also noted (p.163). While parents tended to under-estimate the emotional effect on the child of the illness state, Burton found that over half the school-age children said that the illness made them sad and many expressed fears concerning it. Many children refused to use the school toilets for fear of the comments from class-mates. Burton commented on the general attitude of shame conveyed to the child, which may have negatively affected his self-image.

Nevertheless, a very positive response to school was noticed and Burton suggested that for a child unsure about his own normality, the advent of school may serve to relieve him of that underlying anxiety (p.168). While intelligence testing indicated that the children with CF were normal in terms of intellectual development, attainment tests showed that all the children were retarded in one or more subjects. In looking for answers to this paradox, Burton found a relationship between retardation and the sick child's overall level of anxiety as measured by the Taylor Manifest Anxiety Scale, and between retardation and the CF child's general response to school (p.170). The fact that 25% of parents said that they expected less of their child in terms of school achievement because of the illness must also have influenced the child's own expectations.

Bywater's (1981) study of adolescents with CF found that all 27 interviewed appeared to be well adjusted and without special problems at school; they were not socially isolated and family relationships appeared to be unimpaired. The stage of transfer to an adult hospital was identified as a potential problem, as 14 patients stated that they did not wish to transfer and many of the girls said that they would refuse to do so (p.541). None of the boys felt that there was any problem over the home treatment regimen, but three of the girls felt so strongly about it that they indicated their intention to stop treatment and to leave home when they became 16 years of age. All had a fairly good understanding of CF and only one-third wished to find out more about the illness. Twenty-four said that they preferred not to know more. Only two parents wished to talk to a counsellor - a psychiatrist or a social worker - about their feelings. All but one of the patients said that they could talk to their parents about their illness, although only half had ever done so at any length. It could be added here that the sample related to attendance at a Great Ormond Street Clinic, which could imply an element of self-referral and predominantly middle-class families. While the overall conclusion was that most patients seemed to cope well with their illness and with daily life, Bywater acknowledged that there was some evidence of depression among the girls and that, although they were not socially isolated, they tended not to put themselves in a position where they might feel rejected in that only two went to discotheques or dances.

Sinnema (1984) took three reference groups alongside 64 adolescents with CF - adolescents with asthma, healthy but small adolescents and normal healthy controls. At a younger age CF adolescents were found to show a delay in 'dating and mating' and to be less independent in handling social conflicts and managing their own body hygiene. There were no differences in the formation of ideals and the development of abstract ideas, and CF patients were found to be surprisingly optimistic about their personal future happiness in spite of possible setbacks.

A similarly positive conclusion was reached by Kellerman et al (1980) in their study comparing healthy and chronically ill adolescents for measures of anxiety, self-esteem and perception of control in relation to health. Both CF and diabetic adolescents scored higher than others on control, reflecting their responsibility for their own daily care. It was judged that chronically ill youngsters all under-emphasised the disruption caused by their illness, although the CF patients were noted to think more about their condition when they were well.

There is a consistency in these three studies of adolescents suggesting that the young people used denial effectively as a coping mechanism, but there were areas of immaturity related to self-image and sexuality. Girls consistently showed more distress regarding their physical appearance than did boys.

One other early British study is of particular interest as it developed a nursing perpective on the patterns of stress experienced by families caring for a child with a long-term condition. Harrisson (1977) studied a group of parents whose children had Perthes' disease of the hip, a disabling but curable condition, and a smaller group of parents who had a child with CF. The patient career was seen as a concept central to this study, indicating a series of events having a beginning and progressing through definable stages to an end. Perthes' disease was shown to afford predictable periods of stress related to admission, discharge and the periodic X-rays which monitored progress of the condition. Even in such a highly predictable and apparently uneventful condition with a good prognosis, there were marked problems for parents of which staff seemed almost totally unaware. Follow-up care was almost non-existent. The CF study, incorporating 12 families with 15 children, used tape-recorded interviews and, with eight of the families, health diaries. In her analysis of the patient career, Harrisson used the stages already described - warning or threat, impact, adjustment and terminal - and found that the stages tended to overlap and to have variable timespans for individual families (p.61).

The difficulty of probing sensitive areas was demonstrated in this study, where social isolation and negative attitudes on the part of extended families were admitted, while the effect on siblings and on the marital relationship could not be readily elicited. The reluctance to discuss these issues was thought to reflect the potentially stressful nature of such exploration and it was not felt to be justifiable to add weight to these anxieties by probing at interview (p.72). Cull (1974) also commented on the difficulty of interviewing a child with the mother in the room and felt that this was an inhibiting factor when family relationships were being explored (p.147). Harrisson postulated the value of a longitudinal study to increase understanding of stress as it occurs and its redefinition over time.

Further support for a longitudinal study was found in relation to two comments in Burton's study which were particularly illuminating of the dynamics involved in coping with the stress of life-threatening illness. In relation to the behaviour of the child, Burton (p.188) suggested that while he was under strain he was offered a real opportunity to test the strength of the relationships that sustained him. In discussing the grief work necessary for parents, the observation was made that full acceptance came only when some meaning could be seen. A final point of interest was the observation that children who returned regularly to the same hospital seemed to gain strength from continuity of staff and being remembered (p.187). Time and meaning seem to have considerable importance in relation to chronic illness.

There was agreement in the literature reviewed thus far that the major part of the burden of coping with a child with CF tended to be carried by the mother. Bywater's (1981) study of adolescents with CF and their families confirmed this, and rated the depression of mothers caring for a child with CF as higher than that of mothers of normal children and than mothers of adolescents with spina bifida (p.542). Oppenheimer and Rucker (1980) sent out 53 questionnaires to parents of children with CF, asking them about their marital status, the sharing of responsibility for the child's treatment, the ability to meet the treatment needs and whether or not the parents had been able to disucss their feelings about the disease with each other (p 413). Sixteen families did not respond to the questionnaire. The researchers concluded from the findings that proportionately fewer children living with only one natural parent received optimal care at home when compared with children living with both natural parents. A weakness in this study was the fact that the evaluation of optimal or poor care in the home was made by the Medical Director of the Cystic Fibrosis Center and the criteria by which the evaluation was made are not clear. Nevertheless, the case examples illustrated the family tensions surrounding the task of caring for a child with CF and the data suggested that the children living with one natural parent and one step-parent fared less well than children living with both natural parents or with one natural parent only. In considering the implications for social work practice, the writers commented that the assessment of the nature and quality of family relationships was critical. It was felt that the fragility of marriage in the United States was increasingly a factor to be dealt with in considering the total care needed for the optimal management of children with CF, and that new approaches may be needed to meet the particular problems stemming from broken marriages and alternative life styles.

Genetic factors

My contact with the families during fieldwork at this time suggested that genetic factors might have some importance in relation to family stress and CF, and I examined the literature for reference to this aspect of the disease. Both Cull (1974) and Burton (1975) mentioned the factor of inheritance as an added stress which was felt to maximise the parents' emotional distress. Cull found that not all mothers sought out further information and it seemed that they would not welcome information being made available to them (p.327). Only 36% felt obliged to have fewer children than originally intended. It was suggested that the perceived burden of the disease, as distinct from the risk, influenced decisions about future childbearing (p.329). In Bywater's (1981) study, four out of five divorced parents said that the marriage had broken down because of the genetic basis of the illness and three out of four parents who were unhappily married blamed the genetic factor for this. Oppenheimer and Rucker (1980) also noted that in comparison to leukaemia and other life-threatening diseases in childhood, the genetic factor in CF triggered off additional stress and guilt feelings for parents. A mother expressed it best:

> Feelings of guilt are very real with parents of cystic children. After all, we who gave him life are also the cause of his death, so I would ask you to think of the parents as well as the child....
> (Standing, 1987, p.4)

Family dynamics

Recognising from the literature the importance of family stress related to CF, Van Os et al (1985) sent out questionnaires to 159 families who had at least one CF child 18 years or younger; each child was also examined physically and scored on the four categories of activity level, physical status, nutritional status and chest X-rays. Statistical analysis showed that stressful life events were related to the onset and severity of illness. Specifically, four events - marital separation, vacation, a loan of less than $10,000 and divorce - correlated significantly with severity of CF manifested by a course of antibiotic therapy (p.306). Three other factors - a child leaving home, the addition of a new family member and a change in work responsibilities - correlated with X-ray changes. There were limitations to the study, not the least being that the CF patient population was predominantly asymptomatic, but it seemed reasonable to conclude that, by helping families cope with life stress, health professionals may indirectly improve the health of the CF child. The discussion suggested that the causal relationships may involve a very complicated system of social and psychological compensatory mechanisms. From the perspective of a systems-theoretical framework, it could be argued that the link between marital separation, an exacerbation of pulmonary symptoms and an increasing likelihood of divorce demonstrated a positive feedback loop (p.308). The retrospective nature of this study did not allow an analysis of such complex causal relationships. It did, however, draw my attention to the relevance of systems theory in relation to a study of family dynamics and chronic illness.

Venters (1981) identified a gap in the literature in relation to family dynamics in the face of long-term and continuous crisis, and pointed out the weakness of existing studies which revealed only dysfunctional coping and strategies with families succumbing to the hardships of the illness. Her study of 100 families demonstrated again the early reactions associated with shock and anticipatory grieving, but found that these reactions were later replaced by varying degrees of reorganisation and recovery. The majority of families were able to promote the coping strategies of 'sharing the burden' and 'endowing the illness with meaning' (p.292). The highest level of family functioning was found in those families who were able to share the burden of illness, both among family members and with someone outside the family. Those at the medium level maintained extensive sharing within the family but partially closed their boundaries to outside help. A low level of family functioning was characterised by one or few members assuming the total burden of the illness and by confusion in defining the illness situation. The concepts of sharing the burden and endowing the illness with meaning emerged as important factors, justifying their inclusion in the research questions address by this study.

A research team from Toronto assessed the effect of the disease on the family by the use of an inventory of family problems as perceived by the parents and two standardized measures of family interaction (Cowen et al, 1986). The Family Assessment Measure (FAM) looked at seven specific areas - task accomplishment, role performance, communication, affective expression, affective involvement, control, and values and norms. The Family Adaptability and Cohesiveness Evaluation Scales (FACES 11) was used to examine the parents' views on adaptability and cohesiveness. Seventy-eight per cent of the 384 patients attending the clinic were included in the study. The scores of family function were generally in the normal range, although parents of older patients did describe some increase in family dysfunction. The study supported the view expressed earlier by Drotar et al (1981) that the presence of CF did not produce psychopathology in the family, but conceded that CF increased the vulnerability of family members to the stresses of life (p.751). The authors recognised the limitation of the cross-sectional nature of their study, which could camouflage variations in the respondents' status. Again, it was suggested that longitudinal studies would be needed to further explain the complex interaction between the patient, parents, siblings and the progress of the disease.

Siblings

In view of the family focus of this study, it was clearly of interest to explore the experience of healthy siblings of children with CF. There is a relative paucity of research in this area but Craft, working at the University of Iowa, studied the effects on siblings of a hospitalised child. Changes in feeling and behaviour were reported by 123 siblings and their parents using interviews and questionnaires. Siblings reported twice as many changes as did their parents, indicating that parents with an ill child in hospital may not be fully aware of how their well children are faring. Important influences on sibling response were age and the quality of relationship with the hospitalised child; younger siblings were more affected than older (although this finding may be coloured by the fact that younger children were interviewed while older children completed the questionnaire); so too were those whose relationship with the ill child was close. Siblings who had received a limited explanation of the sick child's condition reported more adverse changes than did those who received a full and open explanation or none at all, suggesting that a vague explanation creates anxiety (Craft et al, 1985).

A rigorous study by Breslau et al (1981) looked at siblings of children with cystic fibrosis, cerebral palsy, myelodysplasia and multiple handicaps and compared them with randomly selected children from a cross-section of Manhattan households. A Psychiatric Screening Inventory was completed by the mothers and the proportion of siblings with serious impairment was not significantly different between the two groups. There were fine differences, however, and on four sub-scales - 'self-destructive tendencies', 'mentation problems', 'fighting' and 'delinquency' - siblings of an ill child had higher mean scores, which were statistically significant in the latter three areas. Neither the diagnostic category nor the level of disability of the ill child was found to have a significant relationship to the psychological adjustment of siblings. While reliance on the mother's report could be criticised in this study, particularly with Craft et al's findings in mind, the authors claimed sufficient support from earlier researchers who had used techniques to minimise maternal bias, such as questioning about specific behaviour rather than questions requiring a judgement, to justify the approach. They made the point that there was no single, valid, bias-free approach to the assessment of child behaviour. Clearly, it is a difficult area to research but some of the studies already discussed have explored reactions to having a sibling with CF.

Burton's (1975) subject parents reported that the older siblings of the sick children tended to give in more easily to the sick child, to feel protective and to be less agressive than otherwise. Younger siblings were more likely to feel jealous of attention given to the sick child; more than one was given token physiotherapy to establish parity. Rebelliousness was the problem behaviour most often reported by parents, although they seemed to accept this and the signs of jealousy as natural in the circumstances. A dearth in family communication was again evident in that 53% of mothers had never discussed the illness with their well children. Those who had given explanations had restricted them to a brief description of symptoms, with emphasis on the need for greater overall care. This reticence was reflected in the fact that the well children confined their questions to matters related to treatment rather than to the illness itself (p.190). The finding, however, mirrors that in Turk's (1964) study in which communication between parents and well siblings was impaired. Parents voiced concern about behaviour problems such as "playing sick to get attention", feeding problems and nervousness, but failed to come to grips with the problem, saying "We will give attention to them later" (p.70).

Cull's (1974) study of the siblings was qualified, as was that by Turk (1964), by the fact that her approach was indirect, as she questioned the mother about the response of siblings rather than interviewing children (p.311). Like Burton, she found increased tolerance and caring behaviour in the elder siblings and jealousy in the younger ones. It was reported that the siblings rarely talked to the child about his illness, but Cull pointed out that it was not unknown for older siblings to taunt a CF brother or sister with information about CF. Her suggestion that it could be just as disturbing to be given no information as to be given facts they imperfectly appreciated (p.392) is partially sustantiated by Craft et al's later study. There was an interesting finding that a number of parents admitted that they got more pleasure from their CF child than from the other children in the family and there was a relationship approaching statistical significance to the incidence of reported difficulties with siblings (p.313).

The Canadian study reported that pre-school siblings were more affected by hospitalisation of the CF child than were healthy siblings in older age groups. Some behaviour problems of delinquency, immaturity and cruelty were seen in siblings, reflecting their identification with the physical disability and consequent anxieties of the affected child (Cowen et al, 1986).

There does seem to be some discrepancy in the findings reported. In early studies the dire effect of the grim prognosis of CF on family functioning was emphasised; these have been criticised for their subjective and unsystematic approach, lacking reference to control populations. In more recent studies, children with CF were found to be functioning well and families remained stable. Is it the case, as Drotar et al (1981) suggested, that the improved health of CF children has changed the impact on families so markedly? None of the researchers would claim that having cystic fibrosis leads to psychopathology in either the affected child or other family members. Neither would any claim that there is no emotional impact on the family coping with this illness. There may be a danger, in applying measures which provide objective data amenable to statistical analysis, that the total situation is reduced in a way that obscures fine differences and fails to deepen the insight and understanding of those who are attempting to discern the needs for help and support. From a nursing perpective, it is clear that such families are faced with a formidable health problem; careful study of that problem and its implications for the family as a whole and for individual family members should help to inform the nursing situation. The final aspect of the literature on CF to be examined was that of support.

Cull (1974) and Burton (1975) both looked at the support used by families and Cull concluded that support by the clinic doctor or by the home visiting nurse was more effective than parents' groups. This was not the case with the control (coeliac) group, where exchange of information between parents could be very useful; the problem with the parents' groups for CF families was the potential for confrontation with threatening information. Harrisson (1977, p.70) also found considerable ambivalence in parents' attitudes to the meetings held by the Cystic Fibrosis Research Trust (CFRT), although Oppenheimer and Rucker (1980) observed considerable support and benefit to be gained by those who participated in parents' groups. It may be, however, that the nature and purpose of the groups was different as the CFRT groups tended to focus on information-giving and fund-raising for research more than on psychosocial support.

The grim prognosis was seen to be a crucial factor in the well-being of the families studied by Cull (1974) and indicated a need for special care and help. While mothers of coeliac children did need repeated information about the illness and its treatment, the emotional response was markedly different. Cull's subject group reported very little support from health visitors; 68% had no contact and only 12 out of 50 had been helped by contact with a health visitor. Twenty-six per cent had been helped by a medical social worker but that help had not been easily accessible (p.214). Harrisson's group also gained little support from health visitors, but in Burton's group 53% had been helped by health visitors. They had provided moral support and had taken mothers' misgivings about their children's health seriously. In a number of cases it was the health visitor who pressed for adequate testing and thereby effected the diagnosis of CF (p.30). The point was made by Harrisson (1976) that referral to the medical social worker (MSW) was not practised, due to the fact that the role of the MSW was only partially understood and that many doctors and nurses felt themselves equally competent to meet their patients' psychosocial needs. The ward sister was shown to be the main source of information and the person who would have acted as the referral point to supporting agencies had this been seen as necessary. The fact that staff failed to perceive the parents' responsibilities for their disabled children as stressful underlines the need for greater understanding. Burton concluded that the supportive intervention of a properly trained and helpful third party could be of considerable value to the mental health of all family members (p.222). The whole area of information communication in CF was felt to be a delicate one worthy of further study (Cull, 1974, p.384).

Cull's study indicated the potential value of a home visiting scheme. Parents considered that there was an ongoing need for home visits and that mothers needed opportunities to express their personal feelings about the effects of their child's illness (p.558). The scheme was described by Buchanan (1977) and its value addressed. She stressed the importance of confident, understanding parents to the welfare of the child. The home care sister visited the home after the diagnosis had been given at the clinic. She was able to answer questions, and to give further information and practical help regarding drugs, physiotherapy and diet. A variety of problems were discussed and the paediatric sister could arrange for the family to meet the social worker when necessary. After the initial visits, the frequency of later visits was governed by the degree of parental anxiety, the child's condition or clinic defaulting. This was the pattern of service offered by the home care team when I linked up with them and began working with the families in 1983.

While several studies (Burton, 1975; Cull, 1974; Harrisson, 1976; Venters, 1981; Oppenheimer and Rucker, 1980; Van Os, 1985) suggested a need for involvement of a knowledgeable person outwith the family unit, there is little exploration of the kind of skills that are required for this complex and sensitive work. The literature review thus far presented a picture - albeit at times a confusing one - of the effect of CF on the child and the family, but it did not provide any kind of theoretical framework which might guide practice. In order to develop a fuller understanding of the subject it was necessary to study some of the concepts central to the situation, that is, the family, crisis and coping, loss and bereavement.

The family

In view of the manifold psychosocial implications of cystic fibrosis which have been described, it is clear that there is a need to consider the family as well as the affected child. Increasingly, it is being realised that working with an individual is an inadequate approach to health; Caplan (1961, p.133) made this point in relation to mental health and Kew (1975, p.3) argued against the "concentric view of handicap", in which the handicapped child's special needs occupied the centre of the field of vision. The Court Report (DHSS, 1976) emphasised the need to develop a family focus to the care of children. Perlman's (1983) study of home care found that where the resources of the family were over-extended, serious impacts could follow for the dependent person, the family and ultimately for the community (p.8). Wright and Leahey (1984, p.20) spoke of the major conceptual shift that nursing was making from individual to family-centred health care and argued that this approach to care needed to have a solid theoretical base. The following discussion therefore reviews theoretical approaches to family functioning and considers how these inform the study of families caring for a child with cystic fibrosis.

30

Defining the family

A reasonable starting point to the consideration of family life would be to find a satisfactory definition of the family. Westermarck's (1926) classic definition states that marriage is a relation:

> ....of one or more men with one or more women which is recognised by custom or law, and which involves certain rights and duties, both in the case of the parties entering the union and in the case of children born of it. (p.1)

This gives the definition of marriage first place and emphasises its intitutionalised rights and duties. Thus it is placed beyond mere biological mating, excluding casual sexual relationships and those which are unrecognised by society.

Hanson (1987), writing in the context of family nursing, defined the family as:

> .... a social system comprised of two or more persons who coexist within the context of some expectations of reciprocal affection, mutual responsibility and temporal duration. (p.7)

This definition consciously includes traditional nuclear families, cohabiting or homosexual couples, "…. and any other group characterized by commitment, mutual decision-making and shared goals" (p.7). Even this loose definition seems however to miss the group which is increasingly evident in modern society, the single-parent family, since a young child cannot be said to be engaging in mutual decision-making with its parent.

Terkelsen's definition (1980) is helpful:

> A family is a small social system made up of individuals related to each other by reason of strong reciprocal affections and loyalties, and comprising a permanent household (or cluster of households) that persists over years or decades". (p.23)

Such a definition allows the inclusion of the various family forms prevalent in society today and puts the emphasis on the attributes of affection, loyalty and durability as essential characteristics of family life (Wright and Leahey, 1984, p.25).

More relevant to our study however than mere definition of family is the vivid description offered by Skynner (1976):

31

The institution of the family stands in a peculiarly central, crucial position. It faces inward to the individual, outward toward society, preparing each member to take his place in the wider social group by helping him to internalize its values and traditions as part of himself. From the first cry at birth to the last words at death, the family surrounds us and finds a place for all ages, roles and relationships for both sexes. Our needs for physical, emotional and intellectual exchange, and for nurturance, control, communication and genital sexuality can all exist side by side and find satisfaction in harmonious relationship to one another. It exists to make itself unnecessary, to release its members into the wider community as separate, autonomous beings, only to recreate there images of itself anew. It has enormous creative potential, including that of life itself, and it is not surprising that, when it becomes disordered, it possesses an equal potential for terrible destruction. (p.7)

This description gives a very full picture of the centrality of family life to human and social development, while allowing that it is not inevitably good in its effects on its members. It is congruent, too, with developments in nursing which increasingly recognise the significance of the family in relation to the health and well-being of individuals.

Systems theory

Study of the family in our day must include a consideration of systems theory. Skynner (1976) suggested that general systems theory presented a new conceptual leap in scientific development, providing a new way of looking at phenomena in their total relationships rather than in isolation from one another (p.382). This viewpoint could be applied as credibly to a study of the universe and the process whereby structural changes showed relationships one to another as to physiological systems in living organisms. One of the principles operative is that living things have limits, or a boundary which separates them from the surrounding world. That boundary allows the passage of certain substances into the organism and the excretion of unnecessary elements. On the psychological level, Skynner argued, the formation and preservation of individual identity similarly requires effective boundaries to ensure sufficient communication to transmit information from one generation to another, while at the same time permitting each individual to select and retain some influences and information while rejecting others (p.6). While individuals are seen to consist of many sub-systems, that is, physical and psychological systems, they are also seen to fit within a series of sub-systems, for example, parent-child dyad, within the larger family system which, in turn, is nested within the larger suprasystems of the community, comprising

32

neighbourhoods, school and other organisational systems. Such a series of interlinking systems is illustrated in Figure 3.

Will and Wrate (1985) used the McMaster model to elucidate the basic principles of the general systems approach to family functioning

1. Parts of the family are related to each other.

2. One part of the family cannot be understood in isolation from the rest of the system.

3. Family functioning is more than just the sum of the parts.

4. A family's structure and organization are important in determining the behaviour of family members.

5. Transactional patterns in the family system are involved in shaping the behaviour of family members. (p.12)

The values underlying such statements have to do with the purpose of the family to foster optimal development of each family member.

Accepting that such a position can be challenged as unrealistic, too global or inappropriate to different sub-cultures, Will and Wrate went on to describe the three sets of tasks which a family has to deal with in its role in the social, psychological and biological development and maintenance of its members. These include:

Basic tasks - those requiring the provision of food and shelter, nurturance, affection and support.

Developmental tasks - those associated with individual developmental stages, such as the move from infancy through childhood, adolescence and adulthood as well as those associated with family stages, such as the beginning of marriage, birth of a child.

Hazardous events - such as those associated with illness, accidents, unemployment". (p.13)

A longitudinal study of families provides an opportunity to observe how caring for a child with cystic fibrosis impinges on the capacity to handle each of these sets of tasks. For example, concern about nutrition may greatly complicate the basic tasks and the impulse to protect a frail child may militate against the

33

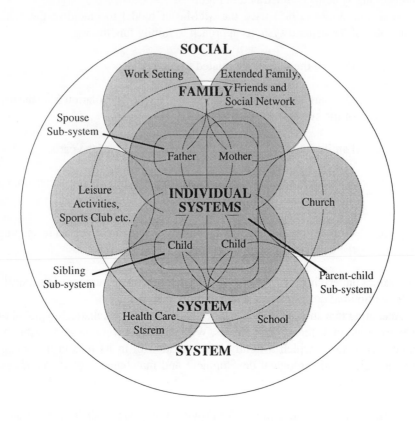

Figure 3
A systems approach to the family
Each member of the family, father, mother and child is a whole system, yet interacts with other family members who are part of the whole family system, The family system interacts within the larger social system which has within it many inter-linking systems. There is a varying amount of interchange across system boundaries

promotion of growth and development. The consideration of hazardous events is particularly relevant since every episode of illness in a child with cystic fibrosis is likely to produce considerable stress for family members, carrying as it does the threat of deterioration.

While accepting that systems theory could not provide a complete predictive theory for family functioning, Wright and Leahey (1984) elaborated the ways in which it could assist understanding of the family as a unit. They defined a system as a 'complex of elements in mutual interaction' and used this as a base for their focus on family interaction in preference to studying family members individually (p.10).

An assessment of a family, then, would include its individual members and its wider relationships. This necessarily involves a recognition of family boundaries. Wright and Leahey pointed out that in family systems, the boundary unit must be both permeable and limiting. Permeability allows the acceptance of outside help but, if it is too permeable, the family's own capacity for coping and decision-making may be compromised and relationships may be disorganised (p.11). Family systems vary greatly in their openness to outside help and it was suggested by Hill (1949), one of the early writers on family stress, that those families which operated a very closed system, isolated even from members of the extended family, were more vulnerable during times of stress (p.270).

The concept of permeability hinges on the idea of the family interacting with its environment. Minuchin (1974) contended that the family must always accommodate to society, in spite of the rapidly changing nature of that society:

Only the family, society's smallest unit, can change and yet maintain enough continuity to rear children who will not be 'strangers in a strange land', who will be rooted firmly enough to grow and to adapt. (p.47)

This view of the centrality of the family for human happiness, individual development and mere survival is now widely accepted. Segal (1983) pointed out that most former critics of the family, including feminists, socialists and scholars, have revised their views and now re-affirm the family as an institution. Nevertheless, the strains and conflicts which led to earlier criticism are still very much with us and family life can be seen to be 'in crisis', with higher divorce rates, fewer births, legal abortion, increasing acceptance of lesbian and gay relationships, of cohabitation, new types of living arrangements and continuing maternal employment. Such rapid societal change must impinge on the dynamics of interaction within families (p.10).

Minuchin (1974) believed that the more flexibility and adaptiveness that society required of its members, the more significant the family became as the matrix of psychosocial development. He proposed a scheme in which the family system had three essential components - structure, development and adaptation to change (p.50). Since Minuchin's work has had a profound influence in family therapy and, consequently, on the development of family nursing in North America, the model which he propounded will be briefly described.

Family structure is defined as "... the invisible set of functional demands that organize the ways in which family members interact" (p.51). The family is seen as a system which operates through transactional patterns. Repeated interactions which define who family members are in relation to each other constitute transactional patterns. The spouse sub-system is vital to the family's functioning and requires of the partners the development of supportive patterns of behaviour - in Minuchin's terms, complementarity and mutual accommodation (p.56). Within the context of the sibling sub-system, children learn how to support, negotiate, co-operate, scapegoat, compete, submit - in short, to experiment with social relationships (p.59).

Family development involves the changes which take place as family members go through varying stages of development and change. This concept is closely related to that of transitions, which will shortly be considered (p.47).

Family adaptation relates also to transitions in that families are required to adjust to internal and external demands for change, yet to provide continuity through a stressful period. The family is transformed over time, adapting and restructuring itself in order to continue functioning. In response to stress, the family has to maintain continuity while making restructuring possible (p.65). A rigid pattern of response may result in dysfunctional patterns of behaviour.

These concepts and their interrelationships facilitate the analysis of family functioning and were used by Wright and Leahey (1984) in their model of family assessment.

Crisis

Crisis can most simply be termed an "... upset in a steady state" (Golan, 1978, p.61) and is usually seen as a turning point in a situation. Hill (1949) defined crisis events as follows:

> ... those situations which create a sharpened sense of insecurity or which block the usual patterns of action and call for new ones. (p.9)

From the work of earlier researchers such as Lindemann, Caplan, Sifneos and Rapoport, Golan (1969) identified four components of an emotional crisis. These were: (1) the hazardous event; (2) the vulnerable state; (3) the precipitating factor;

(4) the state of active crisis. A hazardous event is defined as "... the initial external blow or internal change that triggers a chain of reactions leading to a crisis" (p.390). Golan placed unanticipated hazardous events in three categories: a loss or impending loss of a significant other; the introduction of a new person into the family system; or involvement in a community disaster such as fire or flood. Anticipated hazardous events could either be individual developmental critical stages or transition points such as getting married or retiring.

The vulnerable state has to do with the individual's or family's perception of the initial blow; as a threat to basic needs or to physical or emotional integrity, as a loss of a person or of an ability, or as a challenge. Threat is typically accompanied by feelings of anxiety, loss by depression or mourning and challenge by moderate anxiety mixed with hope, leading to increased energy for problem solving (p.391).

The precipitating factor can be seen as 'the straw that breaks the camel's back'. It is frequently a relatively minor incident in itself but it provides the final link in the chain of stressful events that converts a vulnerable state into a state of disequilibrium, when tension and anxiety have risen to a level beyond the individual's control, this is the state of active crisis.

In a later work, Golan (1981) developed the theme of life tasks which confront all people in the life cycle and referred to these changes as transitions. A transition is defined as "... a period of moving from one state of certainty to another, with an interval of uncertainty and change in between" (p.12). In developmental terms, these periods relate to times of change such as marriage, birth of the first child, the child starting school, children leaving home, the 'empty nest' period, retirement, bereavement. Such experience requires people to cope with feelings of loss and longing for the past, to find new solutions or take on new roles, to handle the feelings of pressure and ambivalence that may be associated with the new situation; adjust to the new solution or role, perhaps with attendant feelings of inferiority or implied criticism from others and to reach a new and different reality (Golan, 1981, p.22). There is considerable agreement that events occurring at the appropriate time in an individual's life cycle rarely precipitate a crisis; events can be anticipated, grief work completed, reconciliation accomplished without shattering the sense of continuity. It is when life events are too sudden or too early that they assume crisis proportions (p.18). The concept of transition seems to apply directly to the experience of a couple learning that their child has an inherited disease; the fact that the disease is life-threatening would perhaps give the event the significance of crisis.

Crisis, according to Caplan (1961):

... is provoked when a person faces an obstacle to important life goals that is, for a time, insurmountable through the utilization of customary methods of problem-solving. A period of disorganization ensues, a period of upset, during which many different abortive attempts at solution are made. Eventually some kind of adaptation is achieved, which may or may not be in the best interests of that person and his fellows. (p.18)

In other words, Caplan's explanation of crisis:

... is what happens when a person faces a difficulty, either a threat of loss or a loss, in which his existing coping repertoire is insufficient, and he therefore has no immediate way of handling the stress. (p.41)

Caplan argued that by some means or other, perhaps due to homeostatic mechanisms, the individual will find a way of handling the situation and that this resolution will be reached within four to six weeks.

The definition used by Mereness and Taylor (1978) adds a further dimension:

Crisis is a state of disequilibrium resulting from the inter-action of an event with the individual's or family's coping mechanisms, which are inadequate to meet the demands of the situation, combined with the individual's or family's perception of the meaning of the event. (p.468)

The concept of meaning was seen in the literature on cystic fibrosis to have some importance in coping with that difficult situation. It would probably be helpful to explore how individuals or families find meaning in the hazardous events they encounter.

In an important early work on families in crisis using a case study approach to analyse family response to separation and reunion, Hill (1949) concluded that, since each family is to a large extent a closed system, the impact of a given situation on its structure will differ in some ways from the impact of a similar situation on another family's structure. The resources which a family brings to meet the situation differ greatly and the definition each family makes of their situation also differs. Some families may treat the situation as a crisis while others regard it as the kind of exigency that all families must face (p.103). In a study of families caring for a very low birthweight baby, McHaffie (1988) again found that stressors became crises in relation to the family's definition of the event. What may be viewed as harmful or damaging by one family may be seen to confer prestige by another. A family's definition of an event, she contended, reflects a combination of its value systems, its previous experience and its coping strategies (p.69).

Coping

A consideration of crisis theory leads naturally to a review of the literature on coping, since the resolution of a crisis requires a response from the individual concerned. Lazarus et al (1974) saw coping as any attempt to master a new situation that appears potentially threatening, frustrating, challenging or gratifying. The concept comes very close to that of adaptation. They make a distinction between situations of differing intensity; in relatively 'low stakes' situations the focus tends to be on deliberate, flexible, reality-orientated efforts at mastery. Conversely, in 'high stakes' situations, where the context is one of strong drive and emotion, the focus is likely to shift to more primitive, less adequate and less realistic efforts at mastery (p.250).

Pearlin and Schooler (1978) defined coping as "... any response to external life strains that serves to prevent, avoid or control emotional distress" (p.3). They surveyed 2,300 adults in Chicago and examined the ways in which they said they had coped with recent stressful events. Three major categories were reported:

1. Seeking to change the situation - by, for example, talking out their situation with those most involved in it, or by adding a new feature to the situation so as to provide new personal resources to assist in coping with it.

2. Redefining the meaning of a stressful situation after it has occurred - by rationalising the experience, saying "It could have been much worse" or "Worse has happened to me before"; a similar tactic is that of positive comparison with others - "I felt I wasn't doing too well till I looked at Fred".

3. Controlling the stress of an experience when it happens - by consciously relaxing and telling oneself to calm down, or by saying to oneself that things will look different in a few days' time.

From their data, Pearlin and Schooler were able to suggest that the most effective coping persons were those who were able to move between these three strategies, that is, they had a broad coping repertoire. Further, those who coped most effectively with stressful life events had three characteristics: they felt very much in control of their own lives; they enjoyed challanges; and they had a strong commitment to self-survival.

Coping should be seen as a dynamic process rather than a static position. Lazarus et al (1974) stated that:

... the coping episode is never a static affair but changes in quality and intensity as a function of new information and of the outcome of previous responses whose implications are appraised. The individual is continually searching, sifting through and evaluating the cues that any situation presents. Some appraisals are rejected and others accepted on the basis of both the steady flow of information and the presence of psychological dispositions that influence the individual's transactions with the environment. (p.260)

The concept of appraisal was further developed by Lazarus. Appraisal is the process by means of which the stakes or potential outcome of a situation, and of the coping efforts adopted by the person to deal with it, are judged or evaluated. Murgatroyd's (1985) discussion helps to clarify the process of appraisal. The primary appraisal stage involves the person in asking of himself such questions as, "Am I OK or am I in trouble?", "Is this a challenge to which I can respond, or a threat?". The questions asked at this stage relate both to the situation in which the person finds himself and to himself, his beliefs, his self-concept, his goals and commitments (p.52). The primary appraisal stage is about the way people see themselves in relation to a given situation.

The stage of secondary appraisal concerns the person's coping repertoire. The question here would be something like, "Do I have the resources to deal with this?". Coping failure at this stage may imply the lack of an appropriate coping response in the person's coping repertoire, a lack of previous experience of such a situation or lack of material resources to enable a specific coping tactic.

Lazarus et al (1974) emphasised that coping represents a transaction between an individual and his environment. The actions and intrapsychic processes that take place in an emotional context certainly depend on the nature of the threat, frustration or potential for gratification. It this were not so, then coping would rarely be adaptive in the sense of preserving the individual reality or making possible the attainment of his goal. Coping can never be assessed, however, without regard to the environmental demands that created the need for it in the first place. Each situation, they argued, must be studied in order to discover how it initiates, shapes or constrains the forms of coping (p.258).

Lazarus et al saw an important gap between experimentation on situational variables and the broader concerns of the study of people coping with environmental events. They questioned the validity of those research projects based on experimental contexts using vicarious (motion picture) threats to college students, from which researchers attempted to generalise to broader contexts of coping responses, coping situations and types of persons (p.286). Ziemer's (1982) study of factors influencing the coping process demonstrated the limitations of a methodology which asked college students to identify which behaviours they engaged in when confronted with a stressful event. Such a retrospective self-assessment is of dubious validity and could hardly be generalised to situations of severe family stress.

This point was elaborated in a careful analysis of the interdependence of cognition and emotion in appraisal and coping. Hamilton and Warburton (1979) considered the range of coping processes and offered four main categories: information search; direct action; inhibition of action; and intrapsychic modes. These processes were seen to have two main functions; one to alter the person-environment relationship, the other to regulate the stress and distress reaction. A person's coping resources were held to vary over time as a result of experience, degree of stress, time of life and the requirements of adaptation associated with different life-styles (p.283). These writers pointed out that every major stressful transaction has its own task requirements. Illness makes different coping demands than taking examinations. It seems important to recognise that while an effective person is likely to cope effectively across a range of circumstances, there may be occasions when the requisite skills are simply not there, or when some hidden personal agenda or psychological deficit intervenes to prevent effective coping.

Children and coping

Rose (1984) attempted to analyse the concepts of coping and vulnerability as they applied to children with chronic conditions. She argued that, while there was much literature on children with chronic health problems, little attention had been given to the transaction between the individual's coping strategies and level of vulnerability and support or lack of support in the environment as determinant of the child's adaptation to living with a chronic condition. Drawing on the work of Murphy (1961), four major aspects of a child's coping resources were identified. These were:

(a)   the range of gratification available to a child;

(b)   a positive, outgoing attitude toward life;

(c)   the range and flexibility of the child's coping devices and defences, that is, being able to delay long enough to plan, being able to fend off the environment, being able to deny for limited periods of time;

(d)   the ability to regress, to retreat to a level of functioning that does not make such acute demands on oneself. (p.178)

41

While a child's behaviour may express coping strategies differently from those observed in adults, the underlying concepts - securing adequate information, maintaining satisfactory internal conditions and keeping some degree of autonomy - hold true from early childhood through the lifespan. Rose then went on to discuss vulnerability, which was seen to have components both inborn and acquired. Vulnerability was viewed as a dynamic continuum along which an individual may move during normal growth and development, with periods of increased vulnerability during times of biologic, social and psychological transitions. In attempting to relate this theoretical framework to clinical practice, Rose described the difficulty a child with cerebral palsy may have in seeking information and demonstrated that this limitation would also reduce his chances of maintaining autonomy. While recent advances in understanding and provision for the needs of cerebral palsied persons went some way towards reducing their vulnerability, there was a clear need for nurses working with such children to be creative in their goal of enabling the child to cope with the environment. Rose concluded:

> Nursing care should focus on minimizing the effect of the vulnerabilities and of maximizing children's coping strategies by providing a predicatable and supportive environment where children can secure adequate information and maintain an appropriate level of autonomy and internal equilibrium. (p.185)

Coping and life-threatening illness

Shady's (1978) review of the literature on coping styles of patients facing life-threatening illness identified the following major responses: denial; depression; anger; suicide; anxiety and fear reactions; psychosomatic complaining; schizoid-type and neurotic-type reactions; regression; dependency; and withdrawal. Denial, in particular, has been recognised to have an adaptive as well as a maladaptive effect when a person is under serious threat. It is recognised that denial can prevent the patient from being overwhelmed and help him make a more gradual transition to an exceedingly difficult situation.

It must, however, also be recognised that denial which produces behaviour which dangerously ignores treatment requirements, or which seriously impedes communication, becomes a maladaptive response. There is evidence, however, that as denial decreases, depression transiently tends to increase. Depression which is turned inwards can lead to thought of suicide; when it is externalised, there may be anger and hostility towards family members and to staff. Anxiety as a concomitant to life-threatening illness was reported by many authors and, as in other threatening situations, it was noted that too much or too little anxiety was found to be maladaptive rather than adaptive. It was recognised that too little fear or anxiety may imply avoidance or withdrawal, two other coping styles frequently related to denial and depression. Shady's conclusion was that the incidence of maladaptive coping techniques, and especially the prevalence of anxiety reactions, supported the need for psychosocial care to accompany physical treatment for patients facing life-threatening illness.

Coping and cystic fibrosis

In a study of 75 families with a CF child, Patterson and McCubbin (1983) tested the proposition made by Hill in 1958 that family life changes, that strains are additive and, at some point, reach a family's limit to adjust to them. A Family Inventory of Life Events and Changes was compiled, listing 171 events and asking families to weight these events on a 0-8 scale, evaluating the amount of adjustment required by the family to cope with the change and whether the adjustment was completed. This was maintained for a six-month period, during which time the child's height, weight and pulmonary function were recorded. The data supported the hypothesis that a pile-up of life changes in a family during a six-month period is associated with changes in the health status of a chronically ill member - in relation to pulmonary function, though not to height and weight. The writers concluded that if the demands of home management were combined with the stress of several life changes, home treatment may be less effective, contributing to a decline in the child's health. It seems important that health workers should recognise that families are frequently adjusting to multiple life changes simultaneously and that this will influence the way the family behaves under stress as much as the single stressor event of which the health care staff may be immediately aware. This paper seemed particularly relevant to the present study because it focused on the care of a child with cystic fibrosis and related vulnerability, stressful events and family resources to first-hand, current family experience.

Developing the work reported above on family coping in relation to a pile-up of events, McCubbin (1984) reported a study which examined parental coping using the Coping Health Inventory for Parents (CHIP), which identifies 80 specific items of coping behaviour and asks parents to record how helpful - on a scale of 0-3 - each strategy is in their experience. Three broad coping patterns are identified in the instrument, the first focusing on family integration, co-operation and an optimistic definition of the situation; the second on social support, self-esteem and psychological stability; and the third on understanding the health care situation. The study found that both mothers and fathers used all three coping patterns and both emphasised family integration. The mother's efforts to maintain social support, self-esteem and psychological stability were negatively related to the child's age, suggesting that as the CF child grows older the mother is less able to use helping strategies in this area. The father's efforts in understanding the health care situation was positively correlated with variables of family income, the greater was the father's tendency to become involved in consultation with the health care staff.

Combining observations from the study and from theory development on family stress, McCubbin was able to identify five interrelated components of adaptation to the stress of having a child with chronic illness. These were:

1. *Intrafamily relations* Family unity in the face of stress is a desired outcome of family coping behaviour and health care intervention. Redefining the family's situation to allow for an optimistic definition of the events is a constructive step in this process.

2. *Social support* Family members acquire emotional support through extrafamilial relationships.

3. *Self-esteem* Improving the self-esteem of the parents can provide them with an increased self-confidence and comfort which, in turn, can facilitate engagement in other coping behaviours and make the parents more able to fit into a change environment.

4. *Health care consultation* Health care providers can serve as advocates, counsellors, co-ordinators, educators and resource persons.

5. *Balance of coping patterns* Families need to balance the extensive care of the CF member with personal investments in themselves as individuals, in the family as a unit and in increasing the understanding of the health care situation.

A similar study was reported by Hymovich and Baker (1985) in which an instrument was developed to measure parents' perceptions of their concerns, needs and coping strategies. Noteworthy among the findings were the facts that over one-half of the parents wanted guidance regarding all aspects of their child's development and about three-quarters of the parents wanted help in understanding their child's condition and its management (p.95). Hymovich and Baker quoted a study by Stein et al (1983) which reported that 74% of parents of children with over 100 chronic conditions said that they had difficulty in understanding their child's disease and wanted further information (p.227). Hymovich and Baker drew the conclusion from this and from their own study that health professionals needed to be available to provide education and anticipatory guidance to these families. By using the assessment tool it would be possible to ascertain the coping strategies which clients were using, to support those that were effective and to recommend alternatives for those strategies that are ineffective. It was also felt that the tool provided a practical means of helping parents express their concerns to health professionals, to realise that they are not the only ones to be facing such problems and that their concerns are seen as important by health professionals.

Both studies demonstrated that an assessment instrument could provide a profile of how the parents of a child with cystic fibrosis were coping at a particular point in time. While the authors visualised that the findings would be utilised in feedback discussions with parents, there was not real guidance on the form such intervention should take. The information yielded also related purely to the parents' perceptions of how the children are coping; while the parents' view is of primary importance, it may not always be accurate.

Loss

Having considered the conceptual frameworks of the family, of crisis and coping, it remains to review some of the vast literature on loss and bereavement since the diagnosis of cystic fibrosis still carries the prognosis of untimely death. The concept of bereavement is briefly considered in general terms, giving way to the main focus of loss, or anticipated loss of a child. Beverley Raphael's (1984) Anatomy of Bereavement provides the background to the analysis since her writing gives comprehensive treatment of most aspects of bereavement and is based on her own research and the work of such seminal thinkers as Freud, Lindemann, Parkes and Bowlby. Illustrations are drawn from autobiographies recounting the experience of bereavement and from research studies.

Raphael (1984) stated that fear or anxiety associated with death was commonly accepted. While this fear had complex underpinnings related to cultural and religious factors, it could be elucidated as a fear of the unknown, fear of pain and mutilation, fear of loss of function, dependence on others, of the annihilation of self and, perhaps most significantly, the fear of loss of those beloved and essential to the self. When the fears became reality and an individual was confronted with the death of a loved one, bereavement reaction followed. This reaction has been systematically studied and described by many workers and is seen to follow distinct stages. It is generally accepted, however, that the stages may overlap and that the bereaved may pass backward and forward among the stages or, indeed, may become locked in one or another (p.20).

The first stage in response to death of a loved one is one of shock, numbness and disbelief. There is often a sense of unreality, of being in a nightmare from which one will awake. Raphael (1984) suggested that the moments or hours of numbness or shutting out may give the ego time to mobilise its resources so that the death and the loss may be dealt with gradually, allowing greater ego control (p.34). With recognition of the loss comes a period of protest or alarm - loud wailing, agitated hand-wringing, anger and restless searching (Black, 1981, p.191). Parkes and Weiss (1983), from their study of bereaved widows, concluded that those suffering from sudden death of a spouse tended to be more at risk of failing to resolve their grief than those who had time to prepare themselves for bereavement, to renew strained relationships and to say farewell (p.52). Pincus (1976), whose comments arose from studies of bereavement as well as from her own experience, suggested that the opposite may be the case. She believed that the severity of grief may be even greater for those who have been able to anticipate the loss, because so much of life may have been absorbed in the joint task of facing death (p.8). Her comments related to the husband-wife relationship but there could be parallels with the parent-child relationship. She pointed out that the involvement with the dying person required almost a complete obliteration of one's personal feelings in order not to deprive both partners of the possibilities remaining in the relationship. In the determined fight for the life of their child, parents may similarly obliterate their own feelings to the point where they are unprepared for the shock of bereavement.

Following the initial stage of shock, there follows a period best described as separation pain (Raphael, 1984, p.40). There is intense yearning, and pining for the one who has been lost, accompanied by restlessness and agitation. Sleep distrubance and anorexia are usual and the bereaved searches for, or finds himself/herself waiting expectantly for the return of, the loved one. This stage was sensitively described by Hill (1974) in her story of a young woman grieving the sudden accidental death of her husband. The feelings of anger - "why did you leave me?" - of searching - having to visit the scene of the accident, spending long hours by the grave - and of withdrawal from those who tried to help are portrayed with a vividness which was explained by the author in a radio interview, "Everything I felt and experienced about D (her lover) dying went into that novel"*.

Marris (1974) described the typical signs of grief as physical distress and a decline in health; inability to surrender the past, such as brooding over memories, clinging to possessions, withdrawal and hostility against others, against fate or

---

*In the psychiatrist's chair" - Interview with Dr Anthony Clare, 30th August 1988.

against oneself. Guilt and blame seemed from the results of a number of studies to vary according to the timeliness of the death; when the death occurred naturally in the fullness of time, grieving was less complicated by guilt feelings than when the deaths were premature and unexpected (p.26).

Gradually, the reality of the loss is accepted and the work of the psychological mourning process commences. The period of fluctuating levels of adaptation was referred to by Green (1985) as "... living on a permanent emotional switchback" (p.127). Hers was an autobiographic account of the illness and death of her husband and of the first year following his death. It is particularly interesting because it gives a searingly honest report of family conflicts, the powerful defence of denial on her husband's part, the reactions of a 3-year old to bereavement and the sense of spiritual conflict as the widow swung between periods of black despair and shining faith. At one stage, there was a plea that people should not expect that after a few months those who have lost someone they love should be 'snapping out of it' when, in actual fact, it was only beginning to sink in (p.111).

During the mourning process the relational bonds have to be undone and the emotions freed for re-investment in life. The young widow quoted by Raphael, a few months after the accidental death of her husband and daughter, said:

> I am so sad. I have lost two parts of myself, of my life, of my whole being. There is a great well of sorrow inside me that will never be dry. Yet somehow, slowly, John and I are going on. We are living and we are going on. (p.50)

One year after the death, she was able to say:

> We are finding our feet ... John and I have our own small quiet world. It's a little family. But we are a family again. (p.59)

One can speak of resolution of the loss as the outcome of bereavement where there is a re-integration into life with new and satisfying attachments valued in their own right.

In pathological bereavement patterns, there is a denial or repression of aspects of the loss and an attempt to hold on to the lost relationship (Raphael, 1984, p.60). Such disturbed patterns may well be seen in a parent grieving the death of a child. The bereaved person is unable to express grief and to review the lost relationship because of the pain involved in relinquishing it. This can lead to chronic grief, with a protracted preoccupation with the lost person.

Children grieve too, though they may show their grief in different ways. Black (p.199) pointed out the need for children to have the experience of the many small

47

losses inevitable in childhood made sense of for them by a parent or other caring adult who could help them to mourn. This, she believed, was a necessary rehearsal for the greater losses which would follow later in life. She commented, too, that coping strategies were learned in the context of the family and suggested that incompleted mourning could produce defences against further losses which would be transmitted to other family members and lead to a rigid family system.

Loss of a child

Raphael (1984) spoke of the pain of untimely deaths, where the sense of being cheated of life and expectations for the future compounds the pain of grieving. She stated:

> Those anticipated years of life will be seen as wasted and lost, and both the dying and bereaved will feel cheated of the relationship that was to be, the experiences that would have been shared. The younger the person who dies, the greater will have been the expectation of the future, and thus, the greater will be the loss that is added to the death itself. (p.24)

Bowlby's (1980) seminal work on loss addressed the question of the different nature of losses as they represent the breaking of different affectional bonds. He suggested that while the pattern of response to death of a child has much in common with the pattern of response to loss of a spouse, there are significant differences in the aftermath of the loss. The sense of loneliness following the death of a spouse is not a prevalent feature following the death of a child. The shattering nature of loss of a child is demonstrated by studies which report an appallingly high casualty rate for individuals and for marriages. Bowlby (1980) cited research which showed the majority of bereaved parents as suffering psychiatric or psychosomatic problems, marital problems and divorce, while siblings of the child who had died showed a high prevalence of emotional disturbances such as school refusal, depression and separation anxiety (p.121).

Two important points emerge from Bowlby's discussion of the loss of a child. One is the conclusion that the outcome of the bereavement:

> ... turns in great degree on the parents' own relationship. When they can mourn together, keeping in step from one phase to the next, each derives comfort and support from the other and the outcome of the mourning is favourable. When, by contrast, the parents are in conflict and mutual support absent the family may break up and/or individual members become psychiatric casualties. (p.121)

48

The other important conclusion is that the pattern of parents' response to a child's fatal illness tends to be shaped during the first few weeks after the diagnosis is made and changes very little thereafter.

Arnold and Gemma (1983) suggested that society failed in its response to the loss of a child. They pointed out that there is no term to describe a parent who has sustained this loss, in the way that a wife becomes a widow, a child an orphan:

> Perhaps parents are not given recognition for the intensity of their loss because a child's death is not fully recognized as a significant loss. It is in living over years that value is attained... The child is not felt to have contributed much in a short life, it is even assumed that a few short years of memories are grieved faster or more completely than many long years of relating. Rather, it is the nature of the relationship and the meaning of the lost member to the survivors that is significant. (p.42)

From their observations as nurses, Arnold and Gemma spoke thus of the particular pain of loss of a child:

> A child's life is precious and each child's death a significant, agonizing blow. Parents grieve forever and live with the memories that they have of their child - each memory vivid and dear, painful and comforting ... The death of a child member affects individual members and the whole family system. There may be a reluctant alteration in family structure and in the members' roles. The strengths and values of the family may be questioned as members turn to or away from the family for support and comfort. (p.26)

The pain of loss of a child must be related to the investment of the parent in the child's life. That investment, an integral part of normal family life, becomes greatly intensified in the joint battle for life which the family undertakes in its nurture of a member with a life-threatening disease. Arnold and Gemma (1983) contended that, on the death of a child, parents experience a shattering loss of self-esteem for the foundation of their significant role as parents has been shaken (p.39).

These observations have considerable implications for the nursing support of families caring for a child with cystic fibrosis. Raphael (1984) pointed out, too, that where death occurs from an inherited disorder, there is an extra element of guilt at having produced a damaged child which is likely to complicate the anticipatory grief and mourning as well as subsequent bereavement (p.270).

Autobiographies show clearly the search for meaning which is part of the process of acceptance. Hill (1974) recounted, through the trauma of unexpected bereavement, a sense of rightness which came and went, a belief that 'he had to die'. In the radio interview she said, "I write seriously to make sense of experience - you take it out of this muddle of emotion and you see a pattern" (see p.82). Koop (1979) described the pain and peace of parents whose son died in a climbing accident:

> It is overwhelming to realize the length and breadth of the tapestry that God has woven around the lives of our family. David's death - the most enormous experience in our lives - was but one stitch in that tapestry, yet everything that happened in the lives of each of us was woven in such a way that many lines of stitches crossed at the moment of David's death. (p.54)

In a moving account by parents of their 25-year old daughter's death with cancer, a sense of meaning was palpable, in spite of the family's rejection of belief in God (Zorza, 1980). Jane was able to prepare for her death by giving presents to her friends and leaving instructions for a party a few weeks after her death, which turned out to be what she wanted, a cheerful thanksgiving. Her mother wrote:

> Before she died, we had talked of how people live on in what they do, in their actions in the memories of those they have influenced. That was how Jane hoped she would live on - and she will. (p.244)

Understandably, those parents who have written of their experience of losing a child are usually those who have survived - and perhaps even gained - through the experience. Michael Kelly (1986) gave a father's account of having a child suffering from a rare inherited metabolic disease which led from delayed development to gross deterioration, loss of consciousness and death by 11 months of age. The stages of adaptation introduced in McCollum and Gibson's (1970) study can be applied to this father's description of a family crisis.

He described his reactions during the protracted prediagnostic stage:

> I didn't care now what was wrong with him, I just wanted to know what it was and to be able to give it a name. Whatever was wrong couldn't be any worse than the anguish of the unknown. (p.47)

In the confrontational stage he admitted that knowing the diagnosis was a big relief, but asked:

How can you accept that your child is going to die? (p. 52)

In relation to the genetic aspects, he had difficulties with the offer of prenatal diagnosis:

> If we went on to abort a child in the future, it implied that we didn't value the life of Simon who was already with us. (p.63)

The sense of blame associated with genetic disease was clearly expressed:

> Even though we were innocent, we still couldn't deny the fact that he had inherited a major genetic disorder from us. Simon hadn't contracted an infection or virus, but was as he was because we had created him that way. (p.64)

After the child had been transferred to a London hospital gravely ill, he was despairing and expressed the reactions of crisis experienced in suicidal thoughts which shocked him but seemed to offer the only real alternative to his suffering and mental anguish, which also produced physical symptoms of aching limbs and tiredness. During the long-term adaptive phase, he commented:

> There is no relief from the daily crucifixion and pain that parents of handicapped children feel. All around are signs that highlight the difference between your child and others. (p.64)

In the terminal phase it is disturbing to note that while the nurses gave an excellent standard of care to Simon, there was always a large professional gap between them and the parents. Only after the death did the ward sister feel able to share her own human feelings and grief about him (p.75).

After the funeral Simon's parents were visited by a couple who had recently lost their teenage son with cystic fibrosis and who had previously lost their three younger children with the same disease. Their readiness to share the grief of the newly-bereaved parents was appreciated and their comment could only have been made by those who had fully shared their suffering - "You can either become a bitter or a better person, but not both. The choice is yours" (p.93).

In the resolution of the bereavement there were problems with the new baby who followed Simon and, for the mother particularly, a profound difficulty in accepting the reality of Simon's handicap, his life and his death. A visit to Lourdes enabled her to come to terms with events and she came home "healed but scarred", and feeling that Simon had led her there in his effort to stop her feeling sorry for herself. The father became involved in self-help groups and he also had a sense of the continuity of Simon's life:

> Simon has given me an experience that has led me into areas that I would otherwise never have seen. He is still turning bad into good. (p.116)

He described the process of adaptation thus:

> The pain never goes, because the loss is permanent, but there is a way in which acceptance of it creeps slowly and by stages into your life. (p.94)

A professional response

The depth of this human experience of loss and bereavement faces nurses and other health care workers with the ultimate challenge in terms of sharing the burden of those who suffer and of seeking to prevent the development of pathological patterns of mourning. Raphael (1984) suggested, however, that there was evidence to suggest that professionals found parental bereavement particularly painful and that the support they gave could be impaired by indentfication with either the mother or the father (p.275). Glaser and Strauss's (1965) study of dying patients and caring staff demonstrated that the death of an infant more than any other could upset the nurse's professional composure (p.232). There are, clearly, difficult issues here which impinge in some extent on the present study although it is not specifically related to terminal illness.

Prior (1981) discussed the complexity of factors which may impinge on an individual family's reaction to the distressing and long-lasting grief of losing a child. Important to the discussion was the problem experienced by modern Western society in dealing with the contradiction of youth and death. Prior suggested that the questions raised by this situation were too frightening to ask, and so the situation was avoided and society refused to acknowledge publicly the right of bereaved parents to mourn their children. The contrast was made with less sophisticated societies, such as an Ethiopian community where a single mother was encouraged to observe a full three-day mourning ritual on the death of her 1-year old twin child. This ritual gave permission for the public expression of feelings of guilt, anger and sadness which positively enabled the mother to adjust to life in a healthy manner after the baby had been mourned. In contrast, bereaved parents in the modern Western world mourned privately and in loneliness. Self-help groups sometimes performed the function formerly provided by traditional mourning rituals.

Responding to the finding that members of the 'helping professions' were frequently seen as unhelpful, Prior suggested specific foci for help in certain circumstances. She emphasised the value of self-help groups and recommended that the therapist should be actively involved in initiating these. The point was made that if the grieving process was not completed by the parents, there was a real risk of the next child becoming a replacement child, with the difficulties for child and for the family unit which that could entail. These were described by Cain and Cain (1964) from their study of disturbed children who had been conceived shortly after the death of another child. These children were filled with fears, could not acquire a separate identity and believed that they too would die in childhood. Prior stressed, however, that the impact of the loss on a family could not be inferred simply from a knowledge of the actual events surrounding the death of their child. As elaborated in the coping literature, each family's reaction is individual in the sense that it takes place against a constellation of background events and is constructed by the individuals concerned on the basis of previous experiences. Hill (1949) also concluded that successful experience with crisis tested and strengthened a family, whereas defeat in crisis was destructive and tended to be repeated (p.12). Prior finally quoted Seligman (1976):

> We are all of us not only victims of our vulnerability but also potential survivors who, at the moment of crisis, are in urgent need of finding within ourselves that vital factor which takes us beyond despair to the point of willing to survive, which requires a capacity to endure pain and guilt and an unshakeable faith in the value of life.

Prior claimed that it was at least part of the task of the caring professions to help victims become survivors (p.326).

Psychosocial transitions

While the concept of loss has an important bearing on the experience of parents caring for a child with cystic fibrosis, it is for them not simply loss in terms of future bereavement but loss of hopes and plans for their child and loss in their total world view. Murray Parkes (1971) wrote of this situation as change in a person's *life-space*, which has been defined as consisting of:

> ... those parts of the environment with which the self interacts and in relation to which behaviour is organized; other persons, material possessions, the familiar world of home and place of work, and the individual's body and mind in so far as he can view these as spearate from his self. (p.103)

A further important concept was that of the assumptive world, "... the only world we know and it includes everything we know" (p.103). This was held to include our interpretation of the past and our expectations of the future. Small changes in life space occur constantly throughout life and can be integrated with experience without necessitating major change or restructuring of the assumptive world, but unexpected major changes such as loss of a job or a body part or a loved one are likely to be seen as major transitions. These are the situations whch Murray Parkes refers to as psychosocial transitions. These are defined as:

> ... those major changes in life space which are lasting in their effect, which take place over a relatively short period of time and which affect large areas of the assumptive world. (p.103)

It would seem from the literature that the concept of psychosocial transitions is highly relevant to the experience of parents learning that their child has a life-threatening inherited illness. A child being part of themselves, and a vital part of their familiar world, means that the threat of loss and the guilt of implication in the cause of the disease constitute a major change in life space.

Summary

Varying accounts have been given of the ways in which such major change affects families caring for a child with cystic fibrosis. Earlier studies described the difficulties faced by child and family, identifying problems of communication as being particularly detrimental to adaptation. Later studies stressed the successful adaptation achieved by many children and their families, and coping strategies of sharing the burden and endowing the illness with meaning were identified. A consideration of the literature dealing with crisis, coping and loss helped to illuminate the problem area, and to provide a theoretical background to the study.

There remained a gap, however, between the studies which focused on psychosocial issues, and the understanding of the entirety of the situation as is required to inform nursing practice. A shift of focus was needed, away from general findings across patient populations to a study of the unique nature of this illness experience from the viewpoint of the families themselves. The aim was not to determine the presence or absence of psychopathology but to develop understanding of how families dealt with the issues which so changed their lives. Inherent in that aim was the intention to study the interaction between family and nurse in order to clarify the role and function of the nurse in what was essentially a long-term commitment. The research strategy to meet these aims is described in the following chapter.

Chapter two:
Research method

It is my view that scientific understanding of the nature of human behavior in relation to health, sickness, crisis states, and tragic life circumstances is highly important to a grounded knowledge base for nursing. (Benoliel, 1984, p.7)

The development of the research methodology is now described, with explanation of the exploratory phase and the development of the research questions. The relevance of the ethnographic method, of qualitative research and a grounded theory approach is critically discussed, taking cognisance of the limitations of the study. This discussion provides the rationale for the adoption of a case study approach and the inclusion of life history interviews. Finally, the progress of the study and related ethical issues are reviewed.

The exploratory phase

The literature search and the early fieldwork clarified the fact that there were questions still to be answered in relation to the experience of families caring for a child with cystic fibrosis. In particular, insight into the effect on the family as a whole and on its individual members was needed. In a search for a research method to guide such an enquiry, I was drawn to the ethnographic approach.

My involvement with the families was first and foremost as a nurse with expert knowledge in the area of cystic fibrosis and with a concern for the welfare of the whole family. This gave me entry to the home and potential involvement in the family system. My assessment of the health and well-being of child and family, exploration of the mother's perceptions of the effect of the child's illness on family relationships, and the recording of full and accurate field notes from the first point of contact provided a kind of pilot phase through which information could be reviewed and the research strategy planned. This was less a pilot study in the strict sense of being a small-scale version of the main study but rather exploratory work which helped me to conceptualise the main areas of concern. Following directly from this conceptualisation came the formulation of the research questions as noted in Chapter 1. The exploratory phase provided rich insights to the family experience and it became clear that an ethnographic approach would be much more effective in providing the data which could inform nursing practice than would a more structural approach. To explain this decision I shall expand on the nature of ethnographic method, qualitative research and grounded theory.

Ethnography

> The ethnographer participates, overtly or covertly, in people's daily lives for an extended period of time, watching what happens, listening to what is said, asking questions, in fact collecting whatever data are available to throw light on the issues in which he or she is concerned. (Hammersley and Atkinson, 1983, p.2)

Ethnography, then, is a form of enquiry which provides the framework for one method of social research. It collects data from a wide range of sources and bears resemblance to the routine ways in which people make sense of everyday life. Its central aim is the generation and testing of theory. Field and Morse (1985, p.21) included observation, interviews, genealogy, demography and life histories in the multiple methods of data collection which may be used by the ethnographer. In support of the usefulness of the ethnographic approach in nursing research they suggested that the knowledge gained was derived from the subject's view of the experience, rather than a view enforced, at least partly, by the researcher, as can be a pitfall where predetermined research tools are used. The detailed descriptive data could be used by practising nurses to help them undertand patients' behaviours. Since users of nursing care were a critical component of any theory of nursing, their beliefs, values and understanding were essential to the development of nursing knowledge (p.22).

Benoliel (1984) wrote of qualitative approaches as:

> ... modes of systematic inquiry concerned with understanding human beings and the nature of their transactions with themselves and their surroundings.   (p.3)

The qualitative data yielded by an ethnographic approach seemed more likely to meet the aim of increasing understanding of the families' experience than quantitative methods. The latter have been widely used in nursing research and have the attraction of scientific tradition. The use of psychometric tests or of questionnaires to large numbers of patients would have given some factual information about the families at a given time, but would not offer deeper understanding of feelings and experience which is a primary purpose of the qualitative approach.

Melia (1982a) discussed the divide in sociology between qualitative and quantitative approaches to the collection and analysis of data:

> The quantitative approach, which takes its lead from the physical and natural sciences, is propounded by those who favour a systematic and objective way of gathering facts about a phenomenon and then, by means of rigorous analysis, arriving at conclusions which, it is argued, are upheld by the data in much the same way as are the conclusions of the natural and physical scientists. The qualitative methodologists, on the other hand, do not place so much emphasis on the idea of predicting human behaviour; rather, they favour the understanding of the behaviour in the tradition described by Weber (1974) as verstehen.   (p.327)

There is probably a similar divide in relation to nursing research, where a tendency exists to use quantitative methods. Melia (1982a) suggested that, as relative newcomers to research wishing to gain academic respectability, nurses may have been attracted to the 'hard' data of survey methods and objective measurements amenable to statistical analysis. She felt, too, that pressures on researchers to produce answers which could form the basis of action may have influenced the choice of methods which could be seen as scientific and legitimate (p.328). Polit and Hungler (1987) believe that there is a growing recognition that both approaches are needed for the advancement of nursing science (p.350). Benoliel (1984), in her argument for the development of qualitative approaches, suggested that people's adaptation of critical life experiences such as chronic illness was one of the broad areas in which this approach offered a valuable expansion of knowledge (p.7).

The important factor in making the decision about the research approach seems to be the subject of the enquiry and the nature of the research question. If there is a direct question to be asked, such as the comparative efficacy of two nursing techniques, for example in catheter care, a quantitative approach is appropriate and the findings can be utilised to inform that area of nursing practice. Alternatively, if one wants to know how having a catheter in situ affects a person's self-image and family relationships, a qualitative approach is required and the findings can be utilised to guide sensitive nursing practice.

The rather simplistic argument above appears to assume that all nursing research must be practice driven or 'applied'. While it is important for any practice discipline to identify problems and attempt systematically to find answers to those problems, it is also important to keep room for 'basic' research which has no more immediate justification than that it may be of interest and potential value to the profession. Melia (1982b) argued strongly in support of basic or fundamental research as being vital in helping nurses explain and understand their day-to-day world of caring (p.12).

Validity

A weakness of the qualitative approach according to its critics is the difficulty of establishing validity, since the gathering of information by one person is clearly open to criticisms of bias. Field and Morse (1985) defined validity in qualitative research as "... the extent to which the research findings represent reality" (p.139). Hammersley and Atkinson (1983) argued that, far from limiting the validity of the study, the involvement of the researcher, once recognised, could be exploited to yield additional insights to the field of study. This was the basis of the reflexivity which they saw as an important strength of the method. They stressed this as the essential character of social research, in that it was part of the world it studied, and the researcher became the research instrument par excellence . While there was no external, absolutely conclusive standard by which to judge the validity of the knowledge gained through this method, it was possible to work with the knowledge gained, recognising that it may be erroneous and subjecting it to systematic inquiry where doubt seemed justified. It was not possible, they argued, to make the researcher "... a neutral vessel of cultural experience" (p.14). This was an important factor in the choice of research method as it fully capitalised the opportunity to develop a nursing perspective through ongoing involvement with the families.

Sampling

Relevant to the question of validity is the place of sampling in the research design. Hammersley and Atkinson (1983) pointed out that a large, randomly selected sample of cases was not necessarily the most useful approach, and that indeed in ethnography it was unlikely to be appropriate (p.44). One is not looking for representativeness as in statistical sampling but for 'information-rich cases' (Patton, 1987, p.52). Field and Morse (1985) contrasted the selection of subjects for a quantitative study with that for a qualitative approach and stated that in the latter approach the researcher would select 'informants' who were willing to talk and had established relationships of trust with the researcher (p.11). Hammersley and Atkinson (1983) suggested that in the early stages of generating theory it was likely that the choice of cases would not greatly matter, while in the later stages of developing and testing theory it may be of considerable importance (p.45).

The sample in fact demonstrates some homogeneity in terms of social class, the age group and sex of the affected children, and the heath problem with which the family was dealing, yet with considerable variation in terms of the severity of the disease. There is a 'deviant case' in that the diagnosis of CF was later withdrawn from one child; this unusual but by no means unique event sheds its own particular shaft of light on the general situation of a family coping with CF. There is also a 'critical case' in which the downward trajectory of cystic fibrosis and the new hopes and fears of transplant surgery are clearly demonstrated. The other two cases could be classified as 'typical cases', portraying families coping in their own distinctive ways with the 'long haul' of caring for a child with a long-term, life-threatening condition which imposes a considerable burden of care, although the children are reasonably well. This classification of cases is based on the work of Glaser and Strauss (1967) who explained "... the discovery of theory from data systematically obtained from social research"; that is, grounded theory (p.2).

Grounded theory

Ethnography is a method which lends itself particularly well to the generation of theory, as was demonstrated so elegantly by Glaser and Strauss (1968) in their work on the care of dying patients, from which awareness theory emerged. In The Discovery of Grounded Theory (1967) they expounded their strategy for handling data and for providing modes of conceptualisation for describing and explaining behaviour (p.3.). Their central thesis was the fact that the theory explicated was systematically obtained from the data, by inductive analysis, not by logical deduction from *a priori* assumptions. The flexibility of the approach, too, was illustrated by their contention that new perspectives can occur on the final day of study or even later, so that there is an ongoing process of generating theory (p.40). Melia (1987) clearly demonstrated the relevance of a grounded theory approach in her study of the occupational socialisation of nurses. She conducted informal in-depth interviews with student nurses and her analysis of the data provided conceptual categories which described and explained student nurses' experience of work and training. In the view of Hammersley and Atkinson (1983, p.19) it is the function of developing and testing theory which distinguishes social research from journalism and literature.

The issue of research methodology was addressed by Blaxter (1976) in her discussion of the design of her classic study of disability. She accepted the criticism that descriptions of individual interactions without making clear how these are to be regarded as more than individual, and without making known and comparable the methods by which the data was obtained, may indeed be no more than journalism. On the other hand, reliance on pseudo-scientific 'instruments' of written questionnaires or structured 'standardised' interviews, ignoring the variable meanings that may be given to the questions by the respondents, may yield problematic, if not meaningless, data. Her study had a longitudinal design with serial interviews and the findings led her to conclude that the validity of any single point-in-time survey must be held in doubt. Where individuals were in a particularly vulnerable state their responses showed considerable change from one interview to the next (p.248).

There seemed no doubt that the ethnographic approach incorporating a longitudinal design was the most appropriate method for this study of the experience of families dealing with chronic childhood illness. The flexibility of approach, the reflexivity and the potential for theory development pointed to its suitability and relevance. A further decision which was important to the development of the study was the choice of the case study approach.

The case study

> We have no need to be ashamed of case-study work. There is nothing sacred about random-sampling or numbers.   (Silverman, 1989, p.75)

Case study research is intensive observation of a single subject, which may be an individual, a group, or an organisation (Meier and Pugh, 1986). It is a strategy which can utilise qualitative or quantitative data, or a combination of the two. Yin (1981) stated that it had the distinguishing characteristic of attempting to examine a contemporary phenomenon in its real-life context, rather than divorce the phenomenon from its context as experimental design would do, or provide information limited to the past, as a history would do. From his own case study work with organisations and from contributions by other researchers, Yin defended the strategy against criticism of the intuitive nature of within-case analysis and the even less well formulated nature of cross-case analysis. His paper accepted that improvements in case study research were still to be made, but reaffirmed the role of the case study as a systematic research tool, claiming that an acceptable craft had already emerged (p.58). Yin's (1984) book provided many helpful pointers for the novice undertaking case studies, but the emphasis on structure, particularly on the definition of questions and propositions at the outset of the study, did not fit comfortably with the ethnographic approach.

Much earlier Dukes (1965) reviewed the many studies regarded as seminal to the development of understanding of psychological concepts, which resulted from observation or experimental work with one subject (N = 1 studies). Several studies were also cited from psychiatry, notably Breuer's case of Anna O, acknowledged to be foundational to the genesis of psychoanalysis. Lest N = 1 studies should be seen as a product of an era unsophisticated in sampling statistics, Dukes tabulated the frequency and range of topics of 246 papers from psychological journals from 1939-1963 which were based on a single subject. In discussing the rationale for N = 1 studies, Dukes argued that, where uniqueness was involved, a sample of one exhausted the population. There were many other uses for such studies - where complete population generality could be assumed to exist, where dissonant findings allowed rejection of an assumed universal relationship, where the population under study was so sparse that a report of one case was useful for a cumulative record or where the situation was extended in time. Problem-centred research on only one subject could clarify questions, indicate approaches and make a substantial contribution to the study of behaviour. Winnicott's (1978) study of a disturbed young child, The Piggle, is an excellent example of such a contribution.

Dukes concluded with a quote from a statistician (McNemar, 1940):

> The statistician who fails to see that important generalizations from research on a single case can ever be acceptable is on a par with the experimentalist who fails to appreciate the fact that some problems can never be solved without resort to numbers.   (p.361)

This comment reflects the view of Silverman (1989) whose detailed discussion of the qualitative-quantitative distinction in social research emphasised the value of qualitative case study research but argued for academic rigour in dealing with data (p.75). The development of theory-based generalisations was seen as an essential part of a case study approach.

Case study research in nursing is dealt with only briefly in most texts. LoBiondo-Wood and Haber (1986) accepted that it allowed for in-depth exploration of newer or unexplored concepts and that it may provide information that would be unobtainable by other methods (p.148). Although the potential for investigator bias was acknowledged, they saw the usefulness of an approach so closely enmeshed in clinical practice. Polit and Hungler (1987) supported the strength of the case study approach for the depth of insight it offered, but argued that this was also a source of potential weakness because the familiarity of the researcher with the subject made objectivity more difficult. They also made the criticism that case study method lacked generalisability (p.169).

Meier and Pugh (1986), however, argued strongly in support of the case study as a viable approach to clinical research. They observed that the ultimate goal of nursing research, in common with other practice-based professions, was improvement in services provided to clients. Where data expanded and clarified the knowledge base of nursing, and the new knowledge was applied in practice, consumers received the benefits of the profession's scholarly activities. Specifically, in view of the expressed commitment to understanding the whole person and those environmental factors that influenced health status, the case study was seen as a strategy well suited to the individualistic focus, characterising the domain of nursing. I would have to add a rider to that, with which Meier and Pugh may well agree, that increasingly nursing has to recognise commitment to whole families, not just to individuals, and this fact justifies the family-centred approach of the present study. Rationales advanced by Meier and Pugh from their review of the literature included the individualistic focus, the longitudinal perspective, and the facility of case study research for bridging the research-practice gap (p.197). Each of these rationales underpins the present study, making the choice of the case study approach a significant component of the research design.

Participant observation

The ethnographic approach then enabled me to share to some extent by participant observation in the lives of the four families. Participant observation is defined by Polit and Hungler (1987) as:

> ... a method of collecting data through the observation of a group or organization in which the researcher participates as a member. (p.534)

There is a sense in which this definition seems not to fit exactly my role as researcher; I did not live as part of the family group. Gold (1958) gave a useful discussion of roles in sociological fieldwork and commented:

Every field work role is at once a social interaction device for securing information for scientific purposes and a set of behaviors in which an observer's self is involved. (p.218)

He discussed the interplay of participation and observation during fieldwork. Complete participation involved concealment of the researcher's activities while he or she participated fully in the life of the group being studied. This method has been fruitfully used in sociological research such as Whyte's (1943) study of street corner society but the role pretence exerts conflicting demands which may jeopardise observation. Hammersley and Atkinson (1983) discussed the issues surrounding 'complete immersion' in the research setting, illustrating how the researcher's activities may be restricted to those of the group, thus reducing the opportunities to interview people and study settings which require free movement (p.94). In contrast, the complete observer had no contact with those being observed, as when observation through a one-way mirror takes place. Between these two extremes lie a number of ways in which behaviour may be observed with greater or lesser involvement of the researcher.

Melia (1987) described her role in conducting single interviews with student nurses as an observer-as-participant role. According to Gold (1958), this approach calls for a more formal approach than more participative roles and is perhaps open to misunderstanding because of the limited contact (p.221). Participant observation was used by Towell (1975) in his study of psychiatric nursing in which he worked as a member of staff for a year, keeping extensive field notes of incidents and exchanges. Since his identity and research intention was known, his role was not one of complete participation. Gold (1958) suggested, however, that this role required pretence of the researcher much as did the complete participant role, in that informants often considered the researcher as more of a colleague than he felt capable of being. There was a danger, too, of the informant over-identifying with the researcher or *vice versa*, the latter causing the researcher to lose his research perspective (p.221).

Bond (1978) described role conflict which was on occasions intolerable during her participant observation study of communication about cancer (p.73). Part of this conflict stemmed from her nursing background which influenced her reactions to stressful situations as well as the perceptions and expectations held of her by others. My role as home visiting nurse ensured my participation in the research setting through interaction with the subjects; my identity and research purpose was known to the families. My role as observer required disciplined recording of the conversations and incidents which occurred as part of that interaction. It is clear that the reflexivity spoken of by Hammersley and Atkinson (1983) was important, as my influence on the research situation added a dimension relevant to the nursing contribution to care. In some respects this reduced role conflict as I was free to act as a nurse, but it required a level of systematic self-analysis which was difficult to achieve.

Nevertheless, balancing the roles of practitioner and researcher, of participant and observer, caused some discomfort at times. One example was taking notes of a telephone conversation while it was in progress, although the conversation was probably no different from the way it would have been if I had not been studying the situation. This kind of tension is accepted by Hammersley and Atkinson (1983) as inherent in the research approach, in which the researcher is intellectually poised between familiarity and strangeness, and socially between stranger and friend (p.100).

The data took the form of field notes completed after each encounter with a family member, whether during a home visit, at the clinic or in a hospital ward, or an informal meeting at a Cystic Fibrosis Research Trust meeting, or fund-raising event. Telephone conversations were also noted during or immediately after the event. The study demonstrates the use of the case study as a research strategy, in which multiple points of contact with the families were utilised. Documentation was also consulted; the diary kept by a play leader was used in one instance. An interview with the nurse who had been previously involved with one family was an additional source of information. This use of multiple sources of data and different approaches is termed triangulation and is regarded as an important technique in maximising the objectivity of ethnographic research. Hammersley and Atkinson (1983) pointed out, however, that triangulation is not simply the combination of different kinds of data, but more an attempt to relate different sorts of data in such a way as to counteract various possible threats to the validity of the analysis (p.199).

The final methodological note relates to the use of a life history approach to an in-depth tape-recorded interview with each member of three of the families, and the mother in the fourth, towards the end of the period of the study.

Life history approach

The life history was defined by Denzin (1978) as presenting:

> ... the experience and definitions held by one person, one group, or one organization as this person, group or organization interprets those experiences. (p.215)

Becker (1966) described it as a method primarily concerned with a faithful rendering of the subject's experience and interpretation of the world he or she lived in.

There were three reasons for incorporating a life history interview into the case study approach. The first was that my main informant over the five-year period of the study was in each case the mother of the affected child. Since I was keen to gain insight into the perspective of each family member, it made obvious sense to ask to interview each individual. As I wanted to know how the experience had been for each of them, the technique of asking them to recall events and feelings related to cystic fibrosis and its impact on family life seemed a useful approach. The second reason was to add depth to the data already gathered. Since the contacts with the families were in the context of a supportive relationship, in the nature of being 'a knowledgeable friend' rather than a context of research interviews, another approach was needed which could frankly draw out information, thoughts and feelings from the informants. The third reason reflects thinking from Becker's (1978) discussion in which he recommended the life history for those times when an area of study has grown stagnant; by the end of four years of accumulating field notes, it was necessary to take a fresh approach which would suggest new questions and provide re-orientation to the field (p.293).

As part of a longitudinal study the life history has an obvious place. The concept of time, as Denzin (1978) commented, both organises and gives meaning to human conduct (p.284). He argued that the life history method could be a most powerful observational and analytic tool. It allowed the construction of a set of explanations that reflected a group's subjective experiences towards a predefined set of events. It facilitated the penetration and understanding of the world as experienced by the subjects.

The combination with the case study approach facilitates a comparison of the subject's definition of the situation with the objective events occurring over time. Becker's (1978) analogy of the mosaic is useful here. He pointed out that each piece added to a mosaic adds a little to our understanding of the total picture; different pieces contribute different things to our understanding. His example related to a 'case history' of Chicago in which different types of data fed in to a study which partially completed a mosaic of great complexity and detail. I would suggest that the field notes of the case studies provide the background of a mosaic, with the life histories allowing us to see more clearly the people in the picture, their individual perceptions and their relationships to one another. In this way they are fulfilling the function claimed for them by Faraday and Plummer (1979) of grappling with the problems of subjective reality and totality of the experience of the subjects.

Progress of the research

In this section there is a summary of the early stages of the research and a discussion of data collection and analysis. The studies began in 1983; my interest in the problems of cystic fibrosis and in the development of paediatric nursing came together almost in a serendipitous way in the arrangement that I would have responsibility for the home visiting of four families caring for a child with CF. With the resolve to undertake research in this area, a general search of the literature relating to CF was made. This, along with the findings of the exploratory phase, helped in the formulation of the research questions. A more specific and structured literature search followed from the conceptualisation of the questions. Access to the homes and hospital clinics and wards posed no difficulty since my honorary appointment legitimated my presence. Nursing and medical staff as well as parents were aware from the outset of my research interest.

Data collection

The unit of analysis was the nuclear family, that is, the parents, the affected child and his siblings. During the course of the study, two older siblings in one family were married, but their spouses were not interviewed. This is not to say, however, that the families were studied without regard to their context and the systems with which they interacted. Support networks were considered and there was direct contact with the schools attended by two of the children.

Fieldwork notes The intitial interview took the form of an assessment of the child's health status, and the Roper, Logan and Tierney (1980) Activities of Living Model was used. There was also a brief exploration of the family structure and relationships. I explained my own role as providing a link between the hospital and home, with a concern for the welfare of the whole family. One of the mothers re-phrased this "like a health visitor for children with an illness" - a definition which I thereafter made use of. I also explained that I worked at the University, teaching on the nursing degree course; that I was particularly interested in cystic fibrosis and the way it affected family life, and hoped to do some research on it. During this initial interview I took notes as my questions were answered; thereafter I carried a diary in case I needed to make myself a reminder, but otherwise did not take notes until I had left the house. These were completed as soon as possible after the visit, but clearly some material must have been lost or slightly changed. It was felt however that this disadvantage was outweighed by the benefit of engaging in natural conversation without the formalising effect of note taking. The entries contained a reference to the sick

66

child's health and identified any current problems. There was also reference to other family members, in relation to health, employment, school or any major life changes.

The same pattern was followed when the contacts were made at the clinic or in hospital. Telephone conversations were most often recorded as soon as possible after they took place; later in the study I frequently took notes during the conversation in order to reduce the material lost and to catch some statements verbatim. In one case, as the child's condition deteriorated and his admissions to hospital became more frequent, telephone conversations frequently took the place of home visits. These conversations were used by the mother to express her feelings and they yielded rich insights to the stress on family members during the final year of the study. Most of the calls were initiated by myself but a parent in three out of four of the families made the call on one or two occasions.

Due to the fact that nursing support was being given concurrently with the research process, there were one or two occasions when the recording of events was less systematic than it would have been if the purpose of the exercise had been solely research. A clinical incident could require intervention at a time when stopping to record notes was not feasible, but the normal strategy was to record the interaction within a few hours of its happening. Clearly it would have been preferable to make the recordings immediately after the event, but this was rarely practicable. The awareness of this methodological weakness had some influence on the decision to tape-record a series of interviews.

Life history interviews The life history interviews were arranged in advance. I explained that the research I had mentioned earlier was near completion and that I would like to speak to each member of the family individually, to learn how cystic fibrosis had affected their lives. In each case permission to tape-record the interview was asked for and given. Confidentiality was assured as it seemed important that each family member should be able to express their feelings with a freedom that may not have been possible if they had felt that the other members of the family would ultimately read what they had said. This seemed necessary in view of the very sensitive areas which were being explored, but it did deny the possibility of going back to the informants for their validation of the material finally presented, as recommended by Denzin (1978, p.248).

It was a particular strength of the study that it was possible to interview children without the presence of their parents, as this has posed a problem to previous researchers (Harrisson, 1977; Cull, 1974). It was decided, however, not to interview the two children of the family from whom the diagnosis of CF had been withdrawn, since the child had never been ill and it seemed unethical to risk raising questions in their minds which may never have been relevant to their experience. Their mother clearly preferred that they would not be interviewed,

67

although she did not refuse permission. The father in this family also was not interviewed; his wife said "Allan is very quiet, you know", and seemed to prefer that the interview would be only with herself.

All members of the other families were interviewed. It was only in one family that each individual was interviewed alone. All the children were interviewed individually but the other two couples shared at least part of their interview time. The interviews were very loosely structured. The intention was to get informants talking about their experience of having cystic fibrosis in the family. Parents were asked to recall the earliest stages of the illness, before diagnosis, and to trace events from then. By this stage in the study the research questions had emerged, and they were alluded to in some way during the interviews, except the question about time. It was felt that a direct question about time might have forced comment in a way that would not be natural, and it was decided to scan the data for spontaneous reference to time. The children were asked to say something about themselves, to 'tell their story' and to recall their first memories associated with CF. My questioning again aimed to cover the areas raised by the research questions, although the interview format was flexible and relatively unstructured. The length of the interviews varied from a little over half an hour with some of the children to over four hours when both parents were involved.

Data collection was completed in late 1988, but because my role in nursing support continues, ongoing involvement with the families makes it difficult to give a clear cut-off point.

This, then, was the process followed in collecting information from the four families. As mentioned earlier, medical and nursing notes were consulted, as well as a diary recorded by a play leader. There was also a tape-recorded interview with the nurse who had visited one family before I became involved. The data are presented in the following chapters, firstly with an outline of each family's experiencing, fulfilling the 'tell it as it is' commitment of this type of inquiry and then with a reflective approach involving cross-case analysis of the questions and issues raised.

Data analysis

Hammersley and Atkinson (1983) made the point that in ethnographic research the data analysis is not an isolated part of the research process but begins at the earliest stage with the formulation and clarification of research problems and continues right through to the writing up phase (p.174). They spoke of a characteristic 'funnel' structure whereby the stages of a research project became progressively focused over time. Through this process a project could be clarified and transformed over the course of the study as the real issues were revealed through ongoing analysis (p.175). Equally, progressive focusing could involve a shift from description to the development and testing of explanations. This process of ongoing analysis is at the core of Glaser and Strauss's (1967) grounded theory approach.

In this study the analysis began, as already described, in the early stages of the project as I assimilated information about cystic fibrosis and the family experience, and tried to focus my thinking sufficiently to formulate the research questions. It continued informally to prompt questions during interaction with family members and more formally when analysis of the tape-recorded interviews was undertaken. The tapes were transcribed by myself and I read through the transcripts several times, highlighting important comments and making margin notes. The editing and interpreting of the interviews and field notes resulted in the family profiles. There was a further period of reflection in which themes and issues were identified and theoretical generalisations were made in relation to the research questions. Further analysis led to the development of theoretical perspectives on nursing which are the focus of the final chapter.

Ethical issues

Polit and Hungler (1987) define ethics in research thus:

> ... the quality of research procedures with respect to their adherence to professional, legal and social obligations to the research subjects (p.529).

Since there were no experimental conditions or treatments involved, the issues relate more to the questions on intrusion of privacy and confidentiality than to the risk of causing harm to the subjects. Nevertheless, in view of the mental and emotional pain involved in dealing with life-threatening illness in children, there was a potential for causing mental discomfort by the use of probing questions. Sensitivity to this hazard guided the questioning during the life history interviews. There were occasions where deeper questioning might have revealed intense conflicts and fears, but it was not felt to be right to do so when there was no way of removing the source of such emotions, that is, the grim prognosis of CF. In honesty, also, I must admit to a sense of my own limitations as a counsellor which made me hesitant to expose emotions in the informant with which I would be unable to give sufficient help. This reveals one aspect of the conflict between the role of practitioner and researcher; perhaps a more dedicated researcher would have squeezed out the greatest possible amount of information in the interests of the study. Nursing research, however, in any case takes place within a professional context in which the well-being of the client is of prime concern and therefore such reticence on my part could equally be seen as maintaining an ethically correct approach to research. A more consistently analytical approach in relation to myself as researcher and practitioner would have maximised the value of the reflexivity of the method

Intrusion of privacy

The extent of contact with a professional person outwith the family system, and the recording of personal information, could be construed as an intrusion of privacy. All the visits were arranged by telephone at times convenient for the mothers and there were attempts to check with them that the level of involvement, in terms of frequency of visits, was acceptable. When the life history interviews were arranged it was explained that identities would be disguised. The response to this from parents tended to be along the lines - "If it'll help someone else, that's alright". One of the affected children generously wished me well in my project.

Confidentiality

True anonymity, in which even the researcher cannot link the data with the informant, was impossible within the research framework. Confidentiality is defined by LoBiondo-Wood and Haber (1986) as protecting the participants in a study so that their individual identities will not be linked with the information they have provided and made public (p.37). This is quite difficult to achieve in case study research. The disguising of personal, social and geographic details can reduce the likelihood of indentification, and the hazards are ameliorated by the fact that the material does not deal with deviant or criminal behaviour, as discussed by Faraday and Plummer (1979) in relation to their work with paedophiles.

In clinically-based research in which the researcher has a long-term relationship with the participants in the study, their interests are safeguarded by the professional, legal and social obligations which underpin professional practice. While I was certainly aware at times of a tension between my role as practitioner and as researcher, I believe that this in no way jeopardised the rights of those who were the recipients of care and the subjects of the research. If anything, the increased interest and motivation stimulated by the research perspective may have enhanced the quality of care provided.

Chapter three:
Family profiles

In introducing the families, I have taken a sequential approach by making use of McCollum and Gibson's (1970) stages of adaptation to organise the information, which covers a five year period. Those stages were: pre-diagnostic; confrontational; long-term adaptive; and terminal, although in this study none of the families reached the terminal stage. Also discussed in Chapter 2 was the work of Will and Wrate (1985) and Minuchin (1974), which was useful in guiding an analysis of the way in which the families interacted and provided for the development and maintenance of their members. The crises experienced by each family over the time of the study are recounted and further aspects of experience which reflect the research questions are touched upon. There is for each family an account of the nursing support given. To a large extent in this chapter I have simply allowed the family members to speak for themselves. Where there are direct quotes the local dialect has been preserved. A more in-depth analysis follows in Chapter 5. A genogram provides a summary of family structure. Figure 4 illustrates the key to the symbols used in the genograms, based on Wright and Leahey's (1984) work on family assessment.

The first two profiles are of the families who have been in the 'long-haul' stage right through the study. The third is of the family who learned three years after the beginning of the study that their son did not in fact have CF. Finally, the family profile of the child whose condition has markedly deteriorated over the period of the study is presented.

The pattern of contacts made with each family is noted in Table 1. This documents the number of interactions with each family and their location.

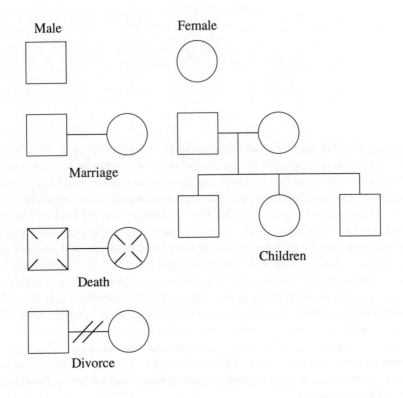

Figure 4
Key to genograms
(Adapted from Wright, L. and Leahey, M. 1984 Nurses and Families p.31)

Table 1

Interactions occurring with each family between 1983 and 1988 according to location.

	Home Visit	Telephone	Ward	Clinic	Taped Interview	Other
Armstrongs	5	3	0	1	1	8
Bruces	9	8	2	14	4	4
Crawfords	18	14	1	8	6	4
Deans	18	36	26	0	3	18
Totals	**50**	**61**	**29**	**23**	**14**	**34**

The names given to the families are fictitious and background information is sufficiently vague to prevent identification. The total number of contacts throughout the study with each family is recorded in Table 2.

Table 2

Total number of interactions with each family

	Total number of contacts
Armstrongs	18
Bruces	41
Crawfords	51
Deans	101

The numbers of contacts with the families reflects the degree of difficulty they were experiencing in coping with the problems related to CF. Interactions were least with the Armstrongs, whose son had been wrongly diagnosed; the greatest number were with the Deans, whose son provided the 'critical case' due to his deteriorating condition.

Home visits were the backbone of the exploration; they provided the most relaxed setting and usually lasted between one and two hours. It is worth noting, however, that Mrs Bruce frequently used the contact during clinic visits to discuss her son's progress and other family concerns; she seemed to find it easier to spend an extra half-hour at the clinic than to make arrangements for a home visit. This possibly reflects the pressure of time experienced by working mothers; most home visits to this family were arranged for evenings. This was the only family however in which clinic visits featured prominently.

With some parents there were encounters in the school setting and there were seven contacts with a child at school for reasons which are explained in the case study. 'Other' contacts mostly occurred within the context of Cystic Fibrosis Research Trust (CFRT)* activities.

---

*The Cystic Fibrosis Research Trust, founded in 1964, changed its title to Cystic Fibrosis Trust in 1992. Its goals are to provide funding for research; support and education. The Head Office is Alexandra House, 5 Blyth Road, Bromley, Kent BR1 3RS.

The Crawford family

The Crawford family lived in a council estate on the edge of Edinburgh. Their house had three bedrooms, one public room, kitchen and bathroom; for many years this accommodated the parents and four children. The outside door was always 'on the latch' and there was a constant stream of callers - neighbours, friends and family. The house was kept clean and adequately furnished, although the garden clearly received little attention. Figure 5 shows family structure in 1983.

Janette and Bill were in their mid-thirties when we met. They married as teenagers, against their parents' wishes. Jan was already pregnant and Dawn was born a few months after the wedding. Bill was a manual worker and there were always financial stresses, but family life was happy. Bill had the habit of going out drinking with his pals at the weekends. Jan seems to have accepted this for the most part as normal male behaviour, although her own father had a considerable drink problem. Jan had two sisters living in Edinburgh, but Bill's family were mostly in England.

Jan described family relationships at that time:

> It was great. But I felt, by the time the kids were off my hands, there was something missing. I wanted another baby. Bill and I had a good relationship and we spoke about it, and we decided that if we were having one, we'd have two, rather than having a big gap and then a baby. Then I had Willie.

The birth of a boy after three girls was a cause for great rejoicing. But from the time he was ten days old Jan was aware that there was something wrong. A diagnosis was not reached until Willie was five months old, and the pre-diagnostic stage was a time of great anxiety.

Pre-diagnostic stage: the parents

The baby was crying a lot and having frequent dirty nappies. When he was ten days old Jan's sister-in-law was admiring the baby and asking if he was good. Jan said "Aye, he's good, but I think there's something wrong wi'im". She remembers Bill looking over, but she signalled to him not to discuss it then - and he never brought the subject up again. Over the next few weeks Jan became increasingly anxious, feeling that nobody was listening to her. The doctors appeared more worried about Jan than about the baby, thinking it was postnatal depression. Jan remembered screaming, "there's nothing wrong wi' me, it's the baby". She called a doctor to the house who had known her since she was a child,

75

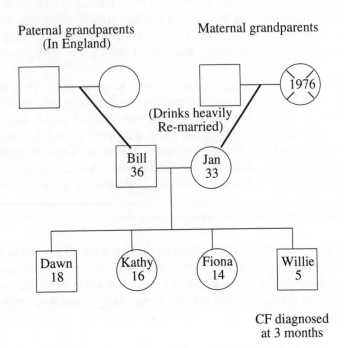

Figure 5

The Crawford family genogram: 1983

and he asked her what she thought was wrong. She answered "I think his stomach's no workin' right, there's a part missing or it's just no working right". Willie was admitted to hospital that day for investigations. Jan said later:

> They should always listen to a mother. I mean, Willie was my fourth, and I never run to the doctor wi' something silly. It's just an instinct that a mother has, and I couldnae get rid o' it.

Bill remembered this period:

> I wasnae even thinking the way she was thinking, like anything serious. If it was something simple, at least we could get it sorted out.

Willie was five months old when the diagnosis was given. Bill admitted that he was really worried by then:

> I could see he wasnae getting better, to me he was getting worse. I wouldnae say nothing to Jan at the time, ken what I felt, you're actually feared to say that. I got to the stage where I didnae want to ask, at the hospital, ken, what was wrong. I was feared they would turn roon' an' say, 'well we reckon we're going to lose him', or something like that.

This avoidance of threatening information typified Bill's reaction to his son's illness.

Pre-diagnostic stage: the siblings

The girls' memories of that five month period were not very clear, but certainly Dawn was aware that her mother was worried. She remembered Jan saying, "He shouldnae have all thae dirty nappies", and how the bottles never satisfied him.

Kathy was just delighted to have a baby brother and used to bring her friends home from school to see him. She remembered how excited her father was when Willie was born, and how he telephoned all the relations. She then recalled coming home to find the doors locked and Willie's pram there, but no-one at home, and a neighbour telling her Willie had been taken to hospital. Her mother tried to explain to her what was happening and she remembered being upset because her mother was upset.

Fiona, at 9, did not understand what was going on. Her parents were aware that, as the youngest, she might feel displaced by Willie, but their anxiety about the baby made it difficult to give her the extra attention they felt she needed. By the time they were faced by the diagnosis they were even less able to respond to

Fiona's needs.

The pre-diagnostic stage was fraught with tension; the parents were not pacing each other in their acceptance of there being a problem and were consequently unable to support each other. The children, although not understanding, were affected to varying degrees by their parents' anxiety.

Confrontational stage: the parents

Jan confessed that her immediate reaction to the diagnosis when suggested to her by the doctor was one of enomous relief:

> I was relieved ... to have a name ... to say to somebody, he's got cystic fibrosis. I mean, I thought Willie was dying. I could have kissed that doctor.

Nevertheless she was shaking when the consultant interviewed them both two days later. She admired the way he told them:

> He was very blunt, but I've got to hear it like that. I've got to be told the truth. He said, he's got a good chance in life because he hasn't had chest infections, but he couldn't guarantee us how long he was going to live. He couldnae give us an age. I appreciated that, to be quite honest.

Of her husband she said:

> It was a blow to Bill, I felt as if I'd two invalids at first. Bill was terrible, drinking ... I couldnae have went to the shops and left Bill to feed him. He'd have fed him, but wouldn't have given him the tablets. (He'd have said) 'What fur? He doesnae need it'. I can understand it now. I couldnae then. I really hated him then.

As far as Bill was concerned, once Willie's weight started going up and he was looking better, everything was fine.

He admitted that he just didn't want to know:

> Looking at him and seeing him getting better, as far as I was concerned he's a'right. For the first few months Jan did it all herself, 'cos I wouldnae accept that he had this disease, an' how dangerous it was.

It took an episode of illness to convince Bill that the problem was not going to go away. At New Year the Crawford household was usually open for all to enjoy a Scottish Hogmanay. A few days before Jan realised that Willie was not well, and she told Bill that she did not want to have the usual party, with all the smoking and kissing going on. At first Bill insisted that he would have his party, but two days before the New Year, he could see for himself that Willie was not well and he told everybody, "the wee laddie's no well, he's got cystic fibrosis and all these germs ...". They both see that as the turning point in Bill's acceptance.

During this period they were visited by a community paediatric nurse who provided a link between the hospital and the home. Jan looked forward to her weekly visits and stored up the questions she wanted to ask:

> ... if it hadnae been for Sister (...) ... I could sit and talk, not just about Willie and cystic fibrosis, I could sit and talk to her about anything and it was mostly about Bill ... because there was times that I was cracking up, but I just couldnae, I wasn't allowed to. I'm no allowed to cry. I used to have my cry on a Friday night, every Friday night, without fail, because that was Bill's night out, aye, an' I'd have a cry, an' I'd feel great after it ... I was like that for a long time.

The genetic aspects of CF clearly intensified the difficulty at this stage. Bill's mother and people in the neighbourhood could not understand how the three girls could be healthy while the fourth child suffered, and the implication was that Bill was not the father. Bill's comments suggest strongly that he could not escape similar suspicions:

> I couldnae understand how Dawn, Kathy, Fiona, there's three I had, there's not a thing wrong wi' them, an' yet, there's Willie ... until they explained to me how it works ... Ken I thought if one person had it, everybody had it, an' that caused problems an' a' ...

Confrontational stage: the siblings

The girls meanwhile were faring as well as they could, not understanding the problem but aware that their parents were unhappy. Dawn expressed it most strongly:

> We were a close family, then something like this. It did change life ... you felt sorry for Willie. It's hard to explain, it did change, it changed a hell o' a lot, from just three of us, then Willie coming along, then something wrong, it was a right let down. But there's how it was, you can't change it ... I really felt sorry for my Mum and Dad but I couldn't say that. There again, whenever they gave him a row, I thought, 'you're a bitch', or if it was

my Dad I'd scream at him, 'leave him alane'. If he didn't have CF and he'd done something wrong, I'd have smacked him for it, but I felt that's a shame, he's got CF, you shouldnae be doing that to him.

Jan reckoned that Dawn blamed her for Willie having CF and said, "Dawn really hated me for years".

Kathy only knew there was something wrong with Willie because her mother was crying and Willie was having to take tablets. She felt they were helped by there being an older girl in their school with CF.

Fiona remembered the rows. She explained:

My Dad wouldnae believe that he had cystic fibrosis, like it was his first laddie and he couldn't take it in. Every time my Mum said he wasnae weel, my Dad would start shouting. That's when I realised what was going on ... my Dad saying there was nothing wrong wi' him and my Mum giving him all they tablets, like who do you believe? ... That was hard, like at night hearing your parents arguing about it ... Like before Willie was born I was the youngest, then when he was born he got all the attention. I thought it was a bit hard 'cos for nine years I got all the attention, then it all stopped.

From the stormy period of confrontation the family gradually moved into the long-term adaptive stage. Jan felt that her belief in God helped her to accept the diagnosis. She admitted that she was angry at first:

Why - when he was so wanted? I couldnae even look at a newborn baby in a pram ... But I thought, well Willie is special, and ... he's there because God knew he'd be looked after in this family, and that's how we've got him ... an' that helped me.

Although they were not Roman Catholics, they took Willie to Lourdes when he was two years of age. She explained that she was feeling so helpless because there was no cure. They had been shown how to help Willie with physiotherapy and tablets, but she wanted to try something for herself. A friend ran a disco to raise the funds, and she, Willie and Bill went together for five days. It was a deeply emotional experience through which, according to Jan, Bill was brought to a more realistic appreciation of the seriousness of his son's condition.

The difficulty this family experienced in coming to terms with the diagnosis is evident. Because they were not travelling together through the transition, the dislocation of relationships affected the whole family. There was little sharing of the burden apart from the support offered by the home visiting nurse. The mother was helped in her acceptance by finding some meaning in the event.

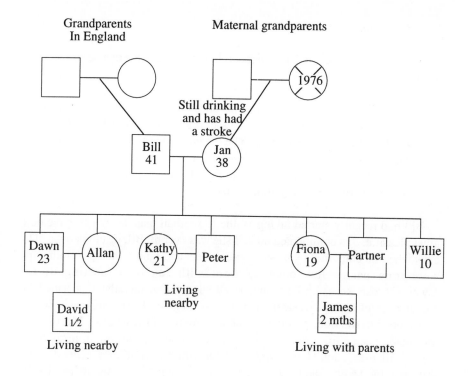

Figure 6
The Crawford family genogram: 1988

Figure 6 represents family structure in late 1988, by which time the family had to a considerable extent adapted to Willie's illness. Willie was 9 years old. His health improved after the early years, which doubtless affected the way the family was coping with the situation.

Long-term adaptive stage: the parents

Bill had long since accepted the diagnosis but admitted to me that he still worried about it:

> I hate when he catches anything because I think ... it's always in the back of your mind, that one of these illnesses is going to put him back in hospital, an' then frae there, it's going to be the end ... In the summer, when we're outside, they (the boys) come up here an' I have the hose out, an' spray them all, an' you look at them all, an' compare them, an' you think, he's thinner, he's no very big, is he getting worse?

Bill had recently started taking Willie to football matches which gave both great pleasure. Jan commented now, if she was ever ill, Bill just took over. The days when he could not be trusted with tablets and ignored the physiotherapy were long past. Just once he went with Jan to a meeting of the Cystic Fibrosis Research Trust and, because it was a social rather than a medical meeting, he felt it was a waste of time and did not go back. He said that he would like more information, particularly about progress in research. Most of his information came from Jan. He was unable to find any purpose or meaning in Willie's illness; "I don't know why, I just don't think it's fair". His general health was good but he had had recurrent back pain for some years, not helped by the heavy lifting he had to do at work.

Jan was the first source of information on CF for all the family. Although she knew that she could now rely on Bill and on Dawn for help, she rarely called on them. She felt that her sisters had never really understood what it meant to live with CF. Since Bill's parents lived some distance away, and her own mother died before Willie was born, she missed any support from grandparents. That may go a long way towards explaining her unqualified welcoming of professional support. CF as a topic was not often discussed among the family, but Jan was always open with the children and attempted to answer their questions honestly. Dealing with Willie's questions was one of her major anxieties. Having shared in earlier years some of her disapointment and hurt in family relationships, I was quite surprised at her response to my question about the effect CF now had on family life. She said:

Aye, it doesnae affect us in any way now, to be quite honest with you. Because I think we've got it all worked out, and I trust Dawn now. Dawn would step into my shoes tomorrow if she had to.

This perhaps illustrates the weakness of a single interview with families coping with chronic illness. Perspectives change with fluctuations in the child's condition, and while during a good spell parents may experience a sense of security and well-being, that equilibrium is fragile. Later in 1988 Willie was ill with a chest infection and Jan became very upset because Bill stayed out late, again failing to give her the support she needed. She walked out the next day in retaliation, but when she came home Willie had waited up for her and Bill said, "You've no got at me, it's your son you've upset". It was almost a week before that breach was repaired, with Jan making the first move. Her own health was not particularly good and Willie worried about her when she had a chest infection or a bout of abdominal pain.

Long-term adaptive stage: the affected child

Willie, at nine years of age, looked healthy, if a little pale. His consuming interest was football and his ambition was to be a professional footballer. He did fairly well at school and enjoyed maths. He had plenty of friends, although they were not among the group who climbed on roofs and caused trouble. In fact he seemed to have more fears than the average boy of his age; he was afraid of the dark and had to have someone staying upstairs with him when he went to bed, he was afraid of lifts and chose to stay at home one year rather than go south with his parents because he was terrified of the train journey. None of this was apparent in conversation and, although his family said that he thought and worried a lot, his response to my questions was different. He said his life was "just normal" and his pals just treated him like a normal pal. When I asked him what he would tell a younger child who had just found out he had CF, he said:

> I'd tell them don't listen to people that call you names, and you just don't think about it and play and do everything, 'cos it doesn't stop you. Just fight it.

The emphasis on 'not thinking about it' was repeated four times during the interview, but the following excerpt suggests otherwise:

> DW I'm wondering if you've ever said to yourself, why me, why should I have CF? What's it all about? Have you ever thought like that?

83

W   No ... just that I was born wi' it, and just cannae help it, so you've got
       it, till maybe they find a cure.

In that simple statement there is absence of guilt or blaming, acceptance of the
situation and hope for the future, surely the product of quite profound thought in
a nine year old.

Willie's health has been better in recent years and the only spell in hospital was
for removal of adenoids. The only admission of concern was with regard to his
weight, which has been static for several months. He said he wanted to "build
himself up". Apparently though there was only one boy in his class taller than
he, so I asked why he wanted to put weight on. His reply perhaps hinted at the
underlying anxiety:

To just build me up a bit, ken, so I can run fast. I can still do that, it just
doesnae bother me, I don't think o' it.

Denial was clearly operating strongly but appeared a useful defence at that time
rather than causing maladaptive behaviour as it did earlier in his father.

Long-term adaptive stage: the siblings

Life moved on for the girls. Dawn married, living in a flat just around the corner
from her parents. She was still very attached to Willie and reckoned that she
would not move further away because of him. She handled situations in a very
similar way to her mother, although she liked to think out her own solutions to
problems. She was very aware of her parents' suffering and told me of the dream
she had recently, in which Willie had died and her parents were so upset that she
gave them her own baby son, just so they would have somebody in the house. She
recognised that her mother was the stronger character and felt that her father
would "crack up" if anything happened to Willie. When she was pregnant she
was offered genetic counselling but said that she did not want to hear about it:

What they'd say I think I probably already know, and if there was anything,
that's because I dinnae want to know.

The family had an excellent relationship with their family doctor and Dawn
said that if there was anything really "bugging her" she would go to him.

Kathy was to be married in the summer, which may have accounted for the
rosy glow with which she seemed to view her family life. She felt that they were
definitely closer as a family and could speak to each other. She admitted that she
"couldn't handle it" when Willie was ill and her mother was upset, but now that
she was spending a lot of time away from home she loved her time with the family

each day:

> I feel as though we should share it wi' my Mum. It doesn't put any more burden on to me, I'm glad my Mum can speak about it ... An' we should help wi' it, because we're his sisters ... if she couldn't get it out of her system wi' us, who could she talk to about it?

Both parents felt that Fiona suffered most through Willie's arrival and illness. She became pregnant while living away from home in a flat, and Jan was only glad that she had come home, away from a crowd who could easily have led her into drug-taking. Of her pregnancy, Jan said, "I think this is Fiona's way of getting out of things'. It'll be something she can call her own". Fiona treated Willie as a healthy wee boy; they fought at times but when she left home he would always ask her when she was coming back, and was the first to know that she was coming home. From her view, the worst thing about Willie having CF was that he would never be able to have children.

Crisis points and the time factor

Having reviewed the way in which the family moved through the stages of adaptation, there remain two specific areas of interest. The first relates to the way in which the family recognised crisis events. In Golan's (1969) terms, the family can be seen to have encountered a hazardous event with the diagnosis of CF and to be made vulnerable by the threat of loss which remains for as long as they have to live with that diagnosis. It can be expected therefore that quite a minor precipitating factor could lead to a period of disequilibrium, that is, crisis. Each member of the family was asked to identify crisis points related to CF in their past experience. The second remaining area of interest is the time factor. In a longitudinal study of the course of a chronic illness, time is likely to be significant. I did not question the families directly on this, but examined the data for references to time. Figure 7 represents a summary of crisis points related to time.

Deaths of known children with CF The first crisis, apart from the diagnosis, identified by most family members related to the deaths of children who had CF. The first was a girl whose sister was in Kathy's class at school, and who was known to both Dawn and Kathy. When she died the whole school was upset, but for Dawn and Kathy the tragedy had the added dimension of bringing home to them for the first time the seriousness of Willie's condition. Dawn remembered meeting Kathy at school in a hysterical state and taking her to the medical room. The teacher there could not explain much, but she did say that as time went on there was better treatment available, which gave Willie a better chance.

Kathy just remembered running out of the school and going straight home: ... because I wanted to be with my Mum. My Mum would understand how I felt ... I said, 'Mum, Jane died last night'. She just picked Willie up from his toys and again she got upset and she was cuddling him, and I knew something was wrong.

Jan remembered cuddling Kathy, and feeling really sorry for her, but not knowing how to cope with it. She pointed out to her that Willie was not so ill as Jane had been. She remembered that her neighbour was in and that she came over to hug Jan, but she pushed her away, saying "I'm alright", although really she was not.

That crisis did carry benefits however in that the sister of the girl who died was able to talk about it, and to come home with the girls and meet Willie; her acceptance seems to have helped the girls and the experience must have deepened their understanding of the situation. Fiona seems not to have been involved in, or very much aware of, this event.

The second death occurred much later, when Willie was seven years old. Michael was several years older than Willie but the families knew each other and the boys were good friends. Bill mentioned Michael's death as having shown Willie how serious his illness was.

Willie himself just made a passing reference to Michael when he was asked if he had any friends at the clinic he could chat to - "Well we had Michael, but he died, he wisnae very well ... just suddenly". He moved quickly on to another subject and his mother said that even now he would walk out of the room if Michael was being talked about. After that she felt that she wanted to protect him from getting close to other CF children.

Kathy did not feel she could cope with going to the funeral, but Dawn went with her mother. She was very upset and when she came home was trying to hide from Willie that she had been crying. When she had to admit that she had been crying, just a bit, for Michael, Willie was alright and then asked a lot of questions about the funeral, and if Michael's parents were upset, and would Michael be happy in heaven? Dawn was deeply upset by this event, to the extent that she could not sleep and spoke to her General Practitioner (GP) about it. She explained:

So I asked - I didnae want to ask but I had to - to make myself feel better - has Willie got it bad? He said, 'Well, he has got it bad but not as bad as Michael had, and touch wood, Willie's been keeping a lot better than Michael did'. I said, 'What's the chances for Willie?'. He said, 'I couldn't really say that, it's not up to me, but Willie's doing really well, he's putting

Figure 7

Stages of the family's experience in adapting to illness related to time and to crisis points

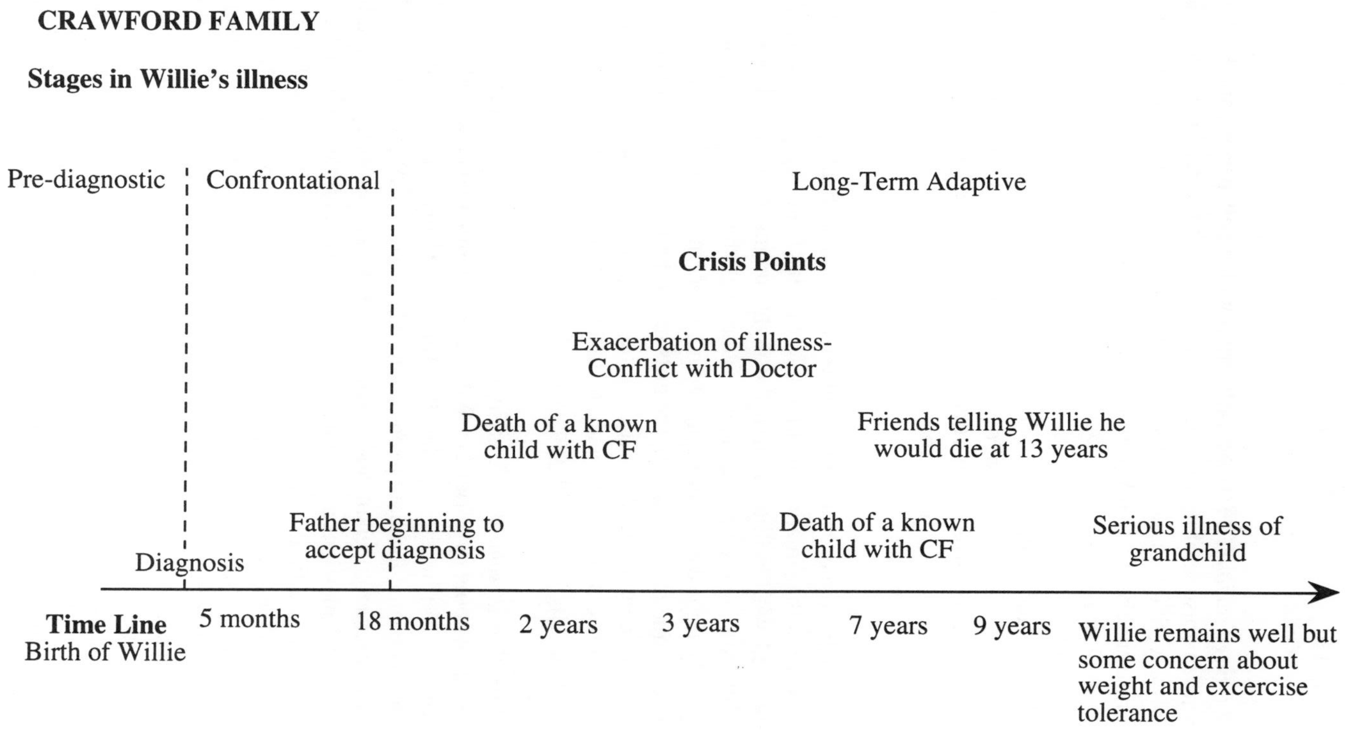

CRAWFORD FAMILY

Stages in Willie's illness

			Long-Term Adaptive			
		Crisis Points				
Pre-diagnostic	Confrontational		Exacerbation of illness-Conflict with Doctor		Friends telling Willie he would die at 13 years	Serious illness of grandchild
			Death of a known child with CF		Death of a known child with CF	
Diagnosis	Father beginning to accept diagnosis					Willie remains well but some concern about weight and excercise tolerance

Time Line
Birth of Willie

5 months	18 months	2 years	3 years	7 years	9 years

on weight, he's never really had to be in hospital for anything, touch wood I hope it stays like that'. He says, 'Willie's a fighter'. Even talking to him made me feel better. He gave me hope.

A bout of serious illness An early crisis which both parents and Kathy mentioned was an episode of illness when Willie was about three years old. He was more wheezy than usual and they had to call out a locum doctor at night, who immediately said that Willie should be admitted. Bill tried to explain that he had cystic fibrosis and was always wheezy, but as he put it:

> As far as she was concerned she was the doctor, we were just parents - but we knew quite a lot by then 'cos we'd seen him a lot worse than that an' heard him better than that ... but she says, 'Well, if you want to build a steam tent in your living room and keep him in it ... and risk going through the night with him'.

On the first occasion the mention of risk made them comply and go to hospital, but when the situation recurred a few nights later, Jan put her foot down. They worked with Willie through the night, taking him in and out of the steamy bathroom, and when the doctor came back the next morning his condition had greatly improved. Jan explained her concern that if she took Willie to hospital every time he was unwell, the girls had to be left with other people and she felt it was like putting four children into hospital. She agreed that she had gained confidence by that time, and said that having Bill helping her made it possible to cope through the night, otherwise she would have agreed to go to hospital.

Taunting at school A crisis mentioned by each member of the family was brought about by a friend of Willie's telling him that he would die by the time he was 13. Willie did not relate the story to me fully, but it formed the background to his comments about people calling him names. Apparently it took him about two weeks to open up and tell his parents what was worrying him; Bill said that he asked questions all round about it, instead of coming right out and asking. Jan said that he finally told Bill when they were sharing a bath together. Bill's reaction was angry, "Tell that little — not to come up here again", but he told Jan about it and she was able to reassure Willie. She told him, "If you staying as well as you are now, there's no way you'll die when you're 13. He just doesn't understand about CF". There were similar incidents around that time and the girls found these extremely upsetting.

Kathy was devastated, feeling that it was just tearing Willie apart. She talked to her boyfriend about it, say she wished she had it, she could cope with it. She remembered how much Willie had been helped by the booklet, 'CF and You', which I had brought to the house just about that time. He had told her, "It's great. It says you can live up to 40, 50, 60, 70". She said:

> His wee face lit up, he feels he doesn't need to listen to anyone else, he's got it in writing. He knows it's not lies. He reads it now. Even when my Mum was telling him it wasn't true what they were saying, he needed something else from someone outside the family, who wasn't reassuring him. I think when he got the book, that really made him accept it.

Fiona's comment on the incident was brief - "You feel like going and hitting them".

Grandchildren's illness   The final crises were not directly related to Willie but to the grandsons. It seems clear, however, that the impact was intensified because of the 'chronic sorrow' - in Olshansky's (1962) phrase - the family already carried. The term was used to describe the natural response of parents to the tragic fact of having a mentally defective child. There seem to be parallels in the experience of parents of a child with CF - the pain of having given birth to a defective child, the prolonged dependence of the child, the demands of treatment and the terrible probability of untimely death.

Dawn's baby, David, contracted meningococcal septicaemia and was admitted to hospital. Jan said:

> I'll never forget that morning, half past three or four o'clock, I just says, 'Why, why us again?'. That really affected me more than Willie having cystic fibrosis. 'Cos I thought, 'What have we done?'.

Mercifully, David made a rapid and full recovery, but the crisis stretched even Jan's resilience. Bill was very supportive and spent a lot of time in the hospital with Dawn, even holding David while blood tests were being taken. Dawn chose not to speak about it, but Kathy mentioned the event, saying that she had gone to the GP because she thought Dawn was "cracking up".

The second such event occurred towards the end of the study. Jan telephoned to say that she was really worried about James, Fiona's baby. He had been in hospital with a viral infection and had not really been well since. He was having loose stools with every feed - "and it smells". Jan felt that everyone was worrying but not saying. The picture was clearly reminding Jan of the early days with Willie; she was not at all an alarmist and I promised to go out the following day, feeling that her hunch was probably right. It was a relief to find that the baby looked fairly well and was gaining weight; the stool she showed me was loose but not offensive. Fiona was sitting in the corner when I went in, sucking her thumb and looking close to tears. She relaxed as we chatted and I talked to James; Jan left us for a while and we talked through the anxieties and pleasures of early motherhood. Fiona said that she had just said to her Mum that day, "It shouldn't be running out him like that, there's something wrong", and her Mum said "I've been thinking that for two weeks now".

There were already arrangements under way for a sweat test as a follow-up to research in genetic mapping from a blood specimen. It seemed justifiable to give some reassurance about James, on the basis of his weight gain and the relatively normal stool, knowing that a definitive answer would be available by the end of the week. The answer was indeed clear; all were relieved, but as Jan said, "We had to have that done". Once the fear was there, it could not be banished without firm evidence.

Time

Time clearly had a negative impact for both parents. Jan had never admitted before how she dreaded Willie's birthdays:

> I think it's maybe because it brings him a year nearer ... D'you ken what I mean? I never show it. I sing 'Happy Birthday' and have a cake and everything, but och, I just get a horrible feeling inside.

Bill had similar thoughts:

> As it goes on, a year, for a healthy person that's just a year, but for Willie it depends on what happened to him that year ... it could get worse for him.

There was a more positive aspect too:

> I'm happy every day wi' Willie. I've had nine good years wi' him, he's still the bairn as far as I'm concerned.

Dawn's perspective was optimistic:

> As each year goes by there's something better coming for them.

Willie's comment showed the courage of so many children with CF:

> I've done that (fought it) for nine years and I'm going to do it the rest.

Having viewed the family's experience from their perspective, it seems appropriate to make a brief analysis of the way in which the tasks of parenting have been handled, and also of the nursing support which has been offered. Will and Wrate (1985) discussed the basic tasks of nurture and provision, the developmental tasks associated with individual development and family transitions, and the task of dealing with hazardous events. The latter has just been considered, but the first two sets of tasks will now be discussed in relation to the Crawford family.

Basic tasks

In spite of family conflicts and financial hardship, Willie was fully provided for in both emotional and physical terms. He was surrounded by the love and affection of all the members of the family. His Christmas and birthday presents were very generous and he was well-clothed and fed. Meeting her son's nutritional needs caused Jan some concern; as a young child he was a very fussy eater and there was always some anxiety about weight gain. His questions were answered honestly and as he matured Willie became highly motivated to improve his nutrition. There was a problem with noctural enuresis until he reached about seven years of age when it spontaneously resolved. Being the youngest and the only boy put him in a privileged position; both parents felt that he was spoiled in the sense of being given preference, particularly over Fiona.

Developmental tasks

The study reflects many of the developmental transitions through which families pass. There was the incorporation into the family of a new baby - with a nine-year gap between him and his youngest sibling; the only boy and one who became the cause of great anxiety and the focal point of much conflict between his parents, with resultant stress for the older siblings. As the confrontational stage gave way to the long-term adaptive stage, events related to CF several times threatened family equilibrium. When the girls were in their early teens Jan felt that they had no respect for "a young Mum" and she was very weary of conflict with them, particularly Dawn and Fiona; she felt that Kathy was the only one who spoke with her. Relationships did improve however and the family restructured itself as the oldest daughter became pregnant and was married, soon presenting Jan and Bill with their first grandson. The wedding was a lavish celebration, putting the family into debt but marking the importance of the event. For the first year or so of their marriage the young couple lived in the Crawford home - an arrangement which was on the whole harmonious as both Jan and Bill found great joy in their grandson. While Kathy's (equally expensive) wedding was being planned Fiona became pregnant. Having been away from her family home, Fiona then came

91

back and her mother was with her during the birth of her baby. Jan continues to give much support and practical help in the care of her second grandson.

Family functioning

The spouse sub-system came very close to breaking down, not because of financial stresses or drinking habits or even violence, but because of Bill's failure to support Jan at the time when she most needed it, in the early stages of Willie's illness. Her deep disappointment in him lasted for some years, but eventually she was able to find some understanding of his reactions and her feelings for him gradually returned. It remained a fragile area, however, in that during a recent bad spell for Willie, Bill still tended to withdraw and go out drinking rather than give Jan the support she needed. One can only be amazed at the strength and resilience of Jan, who has been able to sustain supportive and satisfying family relationships and to maintain continuity through so many turbulent transitions with so little support.

Looking at the family within its wider context, there was little support from grandparents because Jan's mother had died, her father was alcoholic and had re-married; the relationship between Jan and her stepmother was cool. Bill's parents lived too far away to be of particular help, and for a number of years were so sensitive about the genetic aspects of CF that communication was very difficult. Jan's sisters gave little support in the early years, although they have showed more interest in recent years and co-operated with a genetic survey which was being conducted. An elderly next-door neighbour was a close friend and Jan had one or two other friends who gave more support, she felt, than did either family. The staff of the school which Willie attended had previous experience of a child with CF and Jan felt that for the most part the teachers were very helpful. The most recent teacher, however, has been less supportive.

Nursing support

By far the most important aspect of the nursing contribution to care in this case was active listening while Jan talked through some of the problems she was experiencing. As has been shown above, she was dealing with multiple problems with little support, and she made it clear that she appreciated my visits. We were able to explore relationship problems as well as her anxieties about dealing with CF, and in particular with Willie's questions about it. She spoke of the help the previous home visiting nurse had given:

> She just listened. She came every Friday for the first two years. I looked forward to her visit, thought about all the questions I could ask her during

the week. I felt better when she'd left. After about two years she stretched out the visits a bit as I was getting a hold of myself better ... She was a friend as well you know ... she was very fond of Willie, I knew that wisnae right. It must be difficult for the likes of you.

I was able to interview this nurse and ask about the support she had given. She also reckoned that listening had been a big part of her input during the four years she had visited. She rightly described Jan as "the pivot of the whole family" and paid tribute to the admirable care and the affection Willie had been given. There were some regrets about the way the death of the child who had attended the same school as the girls had been handled; since that event it was accepted as being important that the school should be notified as soon as possible after the death, so that staff could be prepared to help other children to cope with their distress. The nurse had been aware of the added problem of drink and some strain on the marriage, but said that she would have felt awkward about asking direct questions concerning family relationships.

The strained relationships and lack of support for Jan were my chief concerns in the early years of contact with Willie and his family. Bill still would not speak about CF, although he obviously thought the world of Willie. Jan said that there were times when she would happily be "up and off". We agreed, however, that this would have a devastating effect on the girls and Willie. I commented that it must have been very hard for Bill to accept that his only son had such a serious disease. She agreed but said that when he was so difficult about it early on, "... something in me died. I just don't feel the same about him any more". Two years later the relationship was much better. Jan said:

> You're the only one I really talk to ... though things are better now with Bill. He helps when Willie's ill, but he still won't talk about it.

She had used physical and verbal abuse after one of Bill's 'binges' and things had been much better after that. It may be that our conversations had some part to play also in helping Jan to gain some insight into the pain behind Bill's refusal to accept Willie's illness and to give support.

On a more practical level, I was able to act as a link person between hospital and home on a number of occasions, checking on an X-ray result which was causing anxiety, relaying information about arrangements for the admission for adenoidectomy, consulting about management of the bed-wetting problem and arranging an appointment with the Medical Social Worker regarding help with the purchase of a bed and later money for a washing machine. I gave moral support at the time the Attendance Allowance was withdrawn, and wrote a supporting letter and helped with the application to have that decision reconsidered, with eventually a successful outcome. I also advised Jan to apply for exemption from prescription charges for her own medication. Specific advice was given with regard to diet; this involved contact also with the dietitian. This particular concern covered the reduction of low-fat milk shakes during the evening while attempts were being made to control the enuresis, the addition of high calorie drinks and snacks to encourage weight gain. There was guidance also for Jan who had been advised to take a high fibre diet because of her diverticulitis. The final area of information-giving was in relation to CF itself, and the provision of information booklets. Helping Jan to be comfortable in her role as primary carer and the source of knowledge about CF seemed the most valuable way of helping the family in this respect.

The Bruce family

The family lived in a surburban terraced house. It had been a council house but the couple decided to buy it, and they proceeded to do a lot of work on it over the years. Hugh and Gill were in their early thirties when we met; Duncan was eight and a half years of age and his sister Shona was six. The family structure is summarised in Figure 8. Both the children had shown positive sweat tests but Shona had no symptoms and was given no treatment. I explained something of my job and my attachment to the home visiting team, which seemed to satisfy Gill who said, "So you're like a Health Visitor for children who have an illness". Duncan's medical history was unusual in that CF was not diagnosed until he was seven years of age, although his mother described him as always being "a semi-sickly child". The pre-diagnostic stage was therefore very protracted, but as his condition was relatively mild, the anxiety seems not to have been as intense as for some parents.

Pre-diagnostic stage

His mother recalled during the life history interview that from the time Duncan was five weeks old he had one chest infection after another. He had been attending a paediatrician:

> ... because when Duncan was born he was thought to have a big head, and he had a large tummy and his pancreas was enlarged, so I attended a clinic ... just to keep an eye on everything.

He was admitted because of a supposed viral infection when he was eight or nine months old. Apart from that the GP had been treating the chest infections. In response to my question, Gill indicated that her anxiety level had not been too high during this time:

> I mean apart from always having a streaming nose and what have you, I just accepted him for what he was ... So he was about four and the chest infections continued and then one summer he had the summer cold as usual and I ended up having six weeks of antibiotics, and the last dose was an adult dose, and a double dose, and I said "No way, this can't go on, there's no way any child should be taking this amount of medicine", and that was when they sent me back to the (local) hospital, and they said at that point that they thought Duncan just had asthma, and this was when they gave him the Spinhaler to see how that worked ... He was about six when he started

95

on that. And then that went on for another wee while, and I thought, "No, this cannae go on".

She insisted on a further referral to the hospital. This time she was shown X-rays which were compared with those taken at the previous visit, and told that it could be one of two things, one of which they could solve, the other "wasn't very nice" and they did not commit themselves at that point. That was when the sweat test came back positive. Gill reckoned that her GP did not know what CF was, because when she went to him for the results of the test he had to get out his medical book and read from it to her. Her first perception of CF was just that it was "a lung disease of children".

Hugh up to this time had not been much concerned:

> I was working all the hours under the sun. I wasnae around nearly as much as what Gill was ... So it didnae really affect me as much as it did Gill. I mean Gill telt me about it but I don't suppose it's exactly the same thing as first hand ... She was annoyed that the doctors weren't getting answers as quick as she wanted them, at times she maybe had a gripe about that at me, but obviously there was nothing I could do and she realised it, it was just a case of her airing her views and getting it off her chest so to speak.

Duncan reckoned that he knew that he had CF "away back, when I was about four or five" but then went on to explain:

> What I remember is, that I went to the doctor's one of the days because my Mum felt that I wasn't quite well. I went to the doctor's and he found out that I had something in my chest ... He contacted the (local) hospital ... and they found out I had cystic fibrosis ... I was about seven when I started going to the Children's Hospital and I've been going there ever since.

When pressed about the timing he repeated that he was about five and, although he could not remember what the doctor had said, he remembered being passed to the Children's Hospital. He did not comment about feeling ill or worried about himself at that time, only that his mother felt that he was not well.

Shona had no recollection of problems before the diagnosis, nor could she remember exactly how or when she first came to know about CF. It seems that during the pre-diagnostic stage in this family, the mother was alone in her concern.

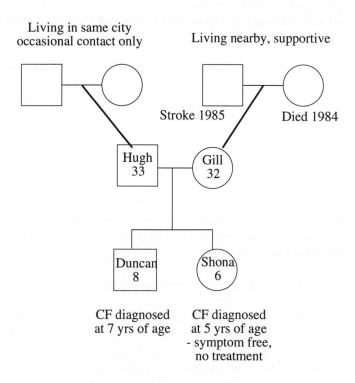

Figure 8

The Bruce family genogram: 1983

On my first visit to the family, Gill spoke only of the relief it had been to them to have a diagnosis after the constant chest infections for which no satisfactory explanation could be given. During the life history interview however, she was more open:

> He (the consultant) told us what it was and how long (inaudible) ... it was the year Hugh was made redundant, and it was just before Christmas that he dropped this bombshell, that both of our children had a lung disease that could be fatal.

She immediately went on to emphasise how Duncan's health had improved after treatment started:

> So in a sense being diagnosed has helped Duncan, not hindered him. So that because we've got a diagnosis, we know what to do, his life is better now since he's been diagnosed ... So if he'd been diagnosed quicker, it'd have been easier on him.

Asked to describe her feelings at the time, she said:

> Very difficult - em - I don't really think I can, just devastated that I was going to lose my wee boy. Why him? You know, why not somebody else's kid, why my son? Why give someone the gift of beautiful big eyes like that, and the gift of the gab and everything, and then destroy him? Something as ridiculous as that - something that nobody can see.

When asked to enlarge on this comment about the invisibility of the illness, Gill said that she felt that Duncan suffered a lot of ridicule because of his hearing difficulty and his frequent coughing:

> If he had a twisted foot or something everybody would see it. I'm not saying they would pity him, which they might do, but they'd have more consideraton for him.

When asked about Shona, she said:

> The thought that Shona had it, just didn't comprehend, because how could someone be as healthy as Shona, do as much as Shona, be so different from Duncan and have something the same as Duncan? It just never occurred

that she had it, and if she had it when was it going to strike? Because surely there should have been some symptoms by that time. And as time's gone on I've just convinced myself, that she can't have it because surely by now ...

Hugh said that he was stunned when they were given the diagnosis, and he too found it difficult to express thoughts and feelings of that time:

Shock is the first one. Concern, worry, if that's the right words - I'm not sure if it is. I didnae want to believe it, once I knew what the disease was, what it potentially does. I just about fell off the chair when he said they just about don't make it to their early teens ... I did ask him - well he explained to us about the chances if we have any more children - the choices of the children ... (inaudible). The immediate thought that came to my mind then was what happens when Duncan gets to that ... Dr A sort of cut me off there - 'We can talk about that later' - and that sort of brought back the point that - well he's not.

(The inference here seems to be that the lack of discussion of Duncan's prospective fertility underlined the probability that he would not reach that stage of development).

Speaking further about his reactions to the diagnosis, he said:

H   I wasnae prepared at all for it. I think both Gill and I knew it was something more than your average 'flus and colds', and - he's also got mild asthma - we knew there was more to it than asthma, we knew within ourselves - I think what we really wanted was just a name put on it - the history behind it, so that we knew, if we could help him any, how to help him because when you don't know what's wrong ...

DW So in that sense, did having a name for it and some treatment, help?

H   Helped tremendously - it did, yea, because the change that we seen in Duncan, the change in weeks, months, as opposed to a long period - the change was phenomenal.

DW It must have been a tremendous mixture of feelings.

H   It was, it was, which is probably what makes it so difficult to talk about. I mean we were relieved in the sense that we now knew what was wrong wi' Duncan ... what we could do, even though it's not that much ... It gave us a bit of relief, well, plus anxiety I suppose in a sense, knowing what cystic fibrosis is and what ...

The genetic implications did not appear to have had a severe impact. Hugh said that it was explained to them that they both had a negative gene:

... and these two negative genes put together is what causes the CF. We've just more or less taken it that in a sense both of us are to blame.

Duncan and Shona appear to have been unaware of the conflicts their parents were experiencing in coming to terms with the diagnosis.

Long-term adaptive stage: the parents

It was about six months after the diagnosis had been given when I first visited this family. Duncan's relatively mild symptoms and the improvement in his general health since the commencement of treatment probably contributed to the relative ease and speed with which the family moved through the confrontational stage into the long-term adaptive stage. As there was no real deterioration as time went on they remained in this stage and the life history interviews reflect the perceptions of each family member five years on. The account at times seems convoluted and tangled, but I have chosen to present the conversations verbatim as they reflect the way in which the family attempted to come to terms with life-threatening inherited illness.

Gill put a strong emphasis on normality. She explained:

Always having Duncan as a semi-sickly child, we've just taken CF into our stride and just kept going ... CF has become part of our life and we've put it there, and just carried on as best we can.

When asked if it was something they talked about as a family, she said:

No, I don't really think so. I mean when I go to the meetings ... I'll come home and we'll discuss it, or if there's any snippets or anything on the TV we'll watch that, but it's not something that we'd come home once a week and talk about or something, it's something that's fitted into the family, it's part of family life.

While he was at primary school a teacher noticed that Duncan was having hearing difficulty, and this became a recurring problem. Gill felt that this

100

probably explained Duncan's rather disjointed speech and at one point commented that they had more problems over his hearing than with CF. She was in no doubt that the main burden of care was on her:

> But then I suppose if they are ill, it's me that's got to look after them, eh, either children, I'm the one that usually has to run to the doctor or to the hospital, though he (Hugh) does do it occasionally ... But the mainstay of the time the responsibility is mine, and if I didn't chase him up, Duncan mainly, say 'Now remember you've got to do it', then nine times out of ten nobody else does, although Shona's quite good and his pal is good.

By this time Duncan was managing his own physiotherapy using the Forced Expiratory Technique; in the early days both parents had learned how to give physiotherapy but Hugh said that Duncan preferred his mother to do it - "He used to grumble a bit, whether I was a bit heavy handed I'm not sure". Gill commented during a home visit in 1985 that she was doing most of the physiotherapy as she was around more than Hugh and she got up more sputum. She felt that their way of coping with CF was keeping family life as normal as possible. In early 1986 we were speaking about school and Gill said:

> There was the problem with the tablets but I've got that sorted out now ... and if he's on antibiotics too I just send them up. His cough does disturb some a bit I know, but really we've had more trouble with his hearing than with the CF. He's not hearing well just now ... Shona's the one that talks about it. She'll say, 'We've got CF'. And (when they were both) at Primary School she used to say, 'Watch my brother, he can't run fast - he's got CF'.

She felt that they were all so used to living with CF that they did not notice Duncan's cough, and that most people who came to the house knew him and what his problems were, and "accepted Duncan for what he is, not for what he's got".

Hugh remained impressed with the improvement in Duncan's health since treatment was instituted. They had been at a Boys' Brigade (BB) camp together and he said:

> ... he ran about that field like any other normal boy, which, before we knew what it was, there was no danger of Duncan going the length of himself.

There had, however, been considerable problems around the BB camp, in that the captain had been unwilling for Duncan to go. Two years previously Gill had telephoned me for help and I arranged for a letter to be sent from the hospital consultant to the BB captain assuring him that there was no reason why Duncan should not go on holiday. That time the camp seemed to go well, but apparently there was still some anxiety if it happened that Hugh was unable to be there as well. Hugh was annoyed that earlier none of the other officers were prepared to learn how to do the physiotherapy - "I suppose just none of them wanted to take the responsibility". He was hopeful that now that it was seen that Duncan did his own physiotherapy without involving anyone else, the staff would be less worried about taking him along. When I asked about Duncan taking his enzymes, Hugh said:

> Em - we've had our troubled times. I cannae see how he can turn round after taking them for all this time - that he's forgotten them. It could be possible for a 13-year old - so involved in other things that the last thing that comes into his head is medicine.

Hugh did not attend the CFRT meetings, although he had been to two of the social evenings. He suggested that this was not so much a decision against going as the fact that he got home from work quite late, but then contended that there might be an element of preference as well as convenience. He rejected my suggestion that parents quite quickly became experts on CF, saying:

> I'd probably like to know an awful lot more than I do, but whether it'd help anything or not I don't know ... whether we've just been more conscious of it I don't know, but there's been a lot more on telly about it. I think since Duncan was diagnosed I've seen about six documentaries that were CF-orientated.'

The emphasis by the parents on normality had its strengths and there was certainly no sign of favouritism or over-protection of Duncan. It may well, however, have raised barriers to communication which ultimately were not in the best interests of any of the family members.

Long-term adaptive stage: the children

Duncan, rather to my surprise as he always seemed cheerful and outgoing when we met, said during the life history interview that he was not very happy; he expressed it by referring to the pictures of smiling and sad faces, and said that his mouth would be straight a lot of the time. Of CF he said:

> It stops you doing a lot of things but as soon as you can fight through, and still manage to do them now and again.

His understanding of CF was quite limited:

> It stops you from breathing because it clogs them up and it means the air, with it (the sputum) growing every second, every second of the time, the air gets crushed more and more so it means you're trying to get it out, some way.

He could not tell me of any other way his body might be affected, and when I asked about his enzymes he was able to relate taking them to stopping diarrhoea. When I asked if that had anything to do with CF he said:

> I don't know. Because I had diarrhoea twice a day, normally you don't need diarrhoea three times a day, so Mum says I've to go down and check to the doctor. So he gave me these tablets that I've been taking for a couple of years now.

Still, when I asked if he thought it was connected with CF, he said:

D   I don't think so. I think that's something different.

DW Is it something you catch, like you catch a cold?

D   I don't think so. Because the thing I heard from Dr A said one time, my Mum had a small tiny wee drop and she carried it on, seeing I was the first-born, I was the one that got the most of it.

DW Right. Actually, your Mum and your Dad both have a wee drop of it.

D   Well **Shona says**, - I don't know whether she's telling the truth or not - that she's got a tiny wee drop of it, but she doesn't need inhalers and that.

DW Uh huh. It doesn't bother her at all, does it?

D   She seems to be like any other ordinary girl.

DW Mm-hm. And would you say you were like any other ordinary boy?

D   Sometimes, but not a lot. Sometimes I don't join in with things that people play, because I don't like the games. Or I find it hard to do that kind of activity.

Recently he had developed a close friendship with a boy who lived close by but he felt that CF put certain limitations on this also:

> He sometimes comes down and stays in my bed overnight, he's asked me if I could go up and stay in his bed, but it really stops me, because his family doesn't know a lot about cystic fibrosis so if something was to go wrong to me they wouldn't know what to do.

When I tried to clarify if he felt a bit nervous about going up to stay with his friend, he said, "It's not me that's nervous, I don't mind going up there, but it's my Mum that's thinking about that."

He was aware that there was as yet no cure for CF, but said he would "hope eventually one of these days, there'll be a cure for it". There was the same approach-avoidance conflict with regard to information that his father had shown. He commented that he did not get time on his own at the clinic to speak about it with someone like the physiotherapist. When I asked if there were any questions he would like to ask me he said, "It's OK, because one of these days I will find out about it. That day'll just have to wait". He insisted that he was quite happy to wait and I did not pursue it further.

Shona was in the ambiguous position of being the well sibling of an affected child, while also knowing that she "had a little bit" of CF herself. She was more forthright in her explanation of CF than her brother:

> I think it's about you get more sputum and things in your lungs, and you can just die of it or something.

She knew that you were born with it and that her parents were carriers, although it did not affect them as an illness. She felt that it did affect her life:

> Yes, because he has to do physio and things and my Mum has to keep on at him, and he can't go and stay anywhere for the night or go to camp

She had some trouble with people in her class at school. When she said in answer to a question from the school nurse that she had a little bit of cystic fibrosis:

> ... all the people in my class sort o' turn against me ... They say, you've got something that might affect me, just keep away, don't want you near us. You should go to a school for other people, not for people like us.

104

Shona laughed when she told me this, saying, "My class is always horrible". It seemed that they were horrible to other people as well and I got the impression that Shona was able to take such comments in her stride. There was evidence though of some disquieting thought:

> I would like to know if it would affect me later. I've not got much of it just now, but later on in life ...

Around this time sweat tests of any doubtful cases were being checked and Shona was clearly hoping that she could be dismissed from the clinic. Duncan's lack of understanding about CF was concerning. I explained about the digestive aspects and the reason for taking enzymes; he listened politely but I felt that he was not eager to try to assimilate the information.

Crisis points and the time factor

The family has been faced with a number of crises in the six-year period since CF was diagnosed. These are summarised below (Figure 9). Some were pinpointed as "crises" or "bad patches" by one or more family members; some were identified from the field notes. Duncan's recurring illnesses followed eventually by the diagnosis of CF constitutes the original hazardous event.

The events related to Duncan were all mentioned by one or both parents during the life history interview apart from the last event, which took place some months after the interviews. They had also been discussed during home or clinic visits. It is worth mentioning also that there were a number of other factors, not directly related to Duncan, which threatened the family's equilibrium during this time. Both parents were made redundant and had a period of unemployment in the first year of the study. Gill's mother died of cancer in 1984 and her father required heart surgery and suffered a stroke the following year. Concern about Duncan's hearing, attendance at ENT clinics and admission for insertion of grommets and for dental extraction all contributed to a pattern of cumulative stress. Gill coped with this with determined fortitude. At a clinic visit in 1984 when Hugh was still unemployed, Duncan was possibly to be admitted for treatment of his otitis media, and Gill's mother had been diagnosed as having cancer with a poor prognosis, I made some expression of sympathy. Gill's response was sharp, "Plenty of people have more problems than I have".

Episodes of illness It was the episodes of illness which caused Gill most anxiety. When Duncan had to be admitted in 1983 there was evidence of guilt and anger. Gill said to me, "That's happened because we haven't been able to give him physio, hasn't it?" I conceded that it would be a factor, and suggested that she

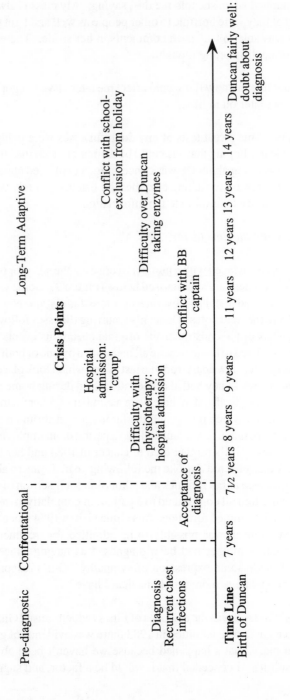

Figure 9

Stages of the family's experience in adapting to illness related to time and to crisis points

use the hospital stay to observe physiotherapy and to be observed by the therapist. She sounded tense and exasperated when the hospital stay lasted longer than expected, and had a sharp disagreement with a staff nurse about it. When he was discharged from the ward she was anxious about the arrangements for physiotherapy, as the doctor stated that it should be given four or five times daily. She questioned that and he reduced it to three or four, and she decided that three times would be manageable as long as her mother could cope with it at lunchtime, as she was working full-time. Over the next six weeks things settled down, a wedge for physiotherapy was supplied and Duncan learned to accept treatment without much complaint.

Duncan apparently took a croup-like illness fairly frequently during early childhood and the hospital admission was brief, seeming not to cause too much upset. These illnesses were, however, identified by Gill as one of her major anxieties.

Difficulty with taking enzymes When Duncan was 12 he became unco-operative about his medication. The capsules which had been given to him to take at school with his lunch were found stowed away in his bedroom. His mother put this down to "a bit of rebellion" and felt it was normal at this age. She was reluctant to involve the Matron as she preferred to trust Duncan. Initially, when arrangements were made for the Matron at school to keep the capsules for him, he did not turn up to take them. When she related it to me, Gill treated the episode philosophically as "just the stage he's at - my friend's wee girl was asthmatic and she was just the same". The problem was resolved and the pattern of calling in on Matron at lunch-time was established. Hugh commented that the difference in Duncan's weight gain after this problem was resolved was remarkable. Previously, it had been a source of disappointment and annoyance to Gill that the school Matron had seemed dismissive of Duncan's problems. From this time onward she clearly appreciated the link with the school which the Matron provided. She was able not only to supervise Duncan but also to ensure that knowledge of his health status and his hearing problem was communicated to teachers.

Conflict about exclusion from group holidays It was in relation to the two episodes of conflict about Duncan joining group activities that Gill telephoned me for support. The question of going to the BB camp was easily resolved by arranging for the consultant to write a letter to the captain, assuring him that there were no health grounds for excluding Duncan. The refusal of the school staff to take Duncan on an overseas trip presented much more difficulty. Gill and Hugh were angry and upset by this decision, and the interview Gill had with the school staff was clearly very fraught. I visited the school and spoke with the teacher concerned and the school doctor. The teacher gave me a courteous hearing but was clearly influenced by the advice of the school doctor, and her position was strongly in favour of the well-being of the whole group in preference to that of one child. Their grounds for refusal were that "it was not a suitable trip for Duncan" because it involved a great deal of travelling; the other factor was that he would have no friends travelling with him and his personality was viewed as something of a problem. This was a surprise since, although both parents had mentioned that Duncan did not have many friends, his cheerful and affectionate manner at home and with adults masked the difficulty he apparently had with his peers. A telling factor which emerged during the lengthy discussions at the school was the common revulsion to sputum. The school doctor said at one point, speaking about Duncan's physiotherapy, "Is it fair to the other children? I mean I could never stand sputum - can you?".

In the end, the doctor's view prevailed and Gill received a letter saying that it would not be possible to take Duncan on the trip. By this time the family had organised themselves to overcome the setback and Duncan was given the compensation of a new keyboard. He was delighted with this and accepted the situation philosophically, but when the objection was originally made he was very hurt, saying that it made him feel that he was just being pushed aside, like rubbish, that he was not wanted. He felt he wanted to be accepted as a normal boy. Gill took up this point when we were discussing it after the event. She said:

> I've never been able to claim attendance allowance or anything for him, but still people don't accept him as normal. He's pig-in-the-middle. It's very irritating.

Her comment illustrates vividly the ambiguity of chronic childhood illness and the frustration experienced when the parents' attempts to maintain normality are obstructed.

Shona could not think of any "bad patch" or crisis, but Duncan related the question to incidents which directly affected him:

> D   When I lose my Ventolin and can't find it, I go all wheezy and everything, I go MAD.

> DW Is that frightening when you go wheezy?

> D   Oh yes, because I really think my lungs are going to give up on me one of these days.

That was the nearest he came to expressing his fears.

The time factor

There were few direct references to time during the life history interviews, but it was very apparent, particularly at the end of the study, that the time element in relation to Duncan's illness was extremely important. At the back of Gill's and Hugh's minds was the knowledge that they had been told not to make plans for Duncan beyond 17 or 18 years and just to take things a year at a time. That they tried very hard to do. For Duncan the time element held a thread of hope - that eventually they would find a cure. Shona was interested in knowing how the disease might affect her later in life. For each member of the family time had a powerful potential influence on events whether for good or ill.

Basic tasks

In terms of the basic tasks, the provision of food and shelter, nurturance, affection and support has been achieved in spite of financial difficulties related to unemployment. The affection was often masked in Gill's case by very brusque commands to the children, but warmth and concern were also there and formed a bedrock of support. When Duncan was asked who or what helped him most to cope with CF, he said:

> Well, my Mum really because she's here in the house, she'd be the one that sometimes remembers me to do my physio, so she's really the one that helps me to get through my life sometimes when I'm in difficulties with it.

Developmental tasks

The developmental tasks of childhood have been completed and the period of adolescence is beginning. Gill is the dominant parent and her determination to keep family life normal ensured that Duncan was not over-protected or favoured at Shona's expense. Her 'no nonsense' approach and Hugh's reserve together ensured that personal feelings were not explored. Conflicts were acted out rather than discussed. This has probably affected Duncan's ability to communicate, which may make for difficulties during the turbulence of adolescence. Problems were also reflected in his peer relationships. Both parents commented at different times that he did not make friends easily, and while the problems with CF and hearing undoubtedly had a part to play, there was also the suggestion from Gill that he was "not enough of a boy. If the teacher told him not to do something, he wouldn't do it". Hugh explained:

> ... he seems to get uptight when they start carrying on and doing things

109

they're not supposed to be doing like all boys sortae do.

It would seem that the combined influences of upbringing, hearing deficit and chronic illness have had a repressive effect on Duncan's nature. Shona, with similar nurture, no hearing problem but a threat of illness, has a bubbly personality and many friends. She apparently bears a very strong resemblance to her mother at the same age.

Gill has shown some awareness of the likelihood of new difficulties as adolescence approaches. When Duncan was 12 she said that he did not ask many questions, but "that's changing, I must look out the leaflets". She said that he knew that it was mostly children and young people who had CF. It seems, however, that Duncan still keeps his questions to himself.

While the pattern of parenting has provided a secure background for childhood growth and development, Gill's firm, almost authoritarian, style may make it difficult to ease the reins a little as Duncan and Shona make their bids for independence.

Family functioning

Within the family structure the spouse sub-system had its conflicts but was sustained by the marital bond and by mutual adaptation. During the interviews we were exploring sources of support; Hugh indicated that Gill was his primary support and also Duncan. Gill named Duncan first, then Shona, and Hugh - "well he brings up the background". The sting was somewhat taken out of this remark by the fact that she was sitting at Hugh's feet hugging his legs while we were talking. Both agreed that the tasks of caring for Duncan were not equally shared, and that Gill carried the major part of the burden. Nevertheless, it was not unusual for Hugh to look after the children on his day off, he would occasionally take time off work to accompany Duncan to the clinic if it was difficult for Gill to do so, and on one of my evening visits he was doing the ironing.

Although Gill rather denigrated Hugh's support at one stage in the interview, when asked what she did if she was feeling upset or worried about Duncan, she said that if there was a medical problem she would "see to it" when she was at the clinic, or else go and see her GP. "Other than that I just shout and scream at Hugh". And it was Hugh that she would talk to about her worries, although she might have gone to her mother when she was alive. She admitted also to being religious, that she prayed - "and get answers back".

This led to my question about meaning, to which she replied:

... I think these diseases have to be man-made some way, so therefore it's bad blood somewhere down the line, previous generations, and we're paying the consequences in later life.

There followed a complex speculation about CF as a modern plague in which something altered the genetic pattern, with AIDS as a parallel though now overtaking CF. This was news to Hugh, who said that he was quite sceptical, but "if it's fated for you it'll happen ... You've just got to get on with life as it happens". He felt that Duncan himself helped him to cope with it - "When you see him coping wi' life, it gives you support".

Hugh was said by Gill to be very quiet, never speaking about anything that worried him. He reckoned that he was good at sitting back and listening, never getting uptight about anything. He also said that CF never raised any barriers between him and Gill, "We've always been a couple that could discuss anything". My impression however was of a coping strategy which operated fairly strongly on denial, in the sense of emphasising the normal and allowing little expression of fears and other uncomfortable feelings. It was an approach which worked reasonably well in maintaining continuity within the family and facilitating adaptation to stress. It is possible, however, that Duncan particularly would benefit from more freedom to express himself and ask questions.

The boundaries within the family were clear and the children were good friends. The family system was relatively impermeable in that there was little reliance on others for help. Gill's parents clearly had been supportive in earlier days and her father still looked after the children sometimes, having made a good recovery from his stroke. Her sister was also very ready to help, but seemed to be regarded as a potential source of help if needed rather than an actual support. A neighbour who had been a good friend and able to help with Duncan was no longer on good terms with Gill. Gill and the children were involved in a church at some distance from their home; there was no evidence of close involvement with people there, although church life was clearly important, particularly for Gill. Relationships with staff at the school were somewhat ambivalent, as has been seen.

Nursing support

In the early contacts with this family there was work to be done in terms of information-giving about CF, its prognosis, and the implications for future fertility. Encouragement was also given with physiotherapy, which was posing difficulties. There was information to be given about a CF holiday which was being planned and a letter of support for an application for Attendance Allowance (which was ultimately refused). It was agreed that home visits were not necessary on a regular basis, and we maintained contact largely through clinic visits and through CFRT activities. After the problem about the school trip there were two further home visits.

Most important was the establishing and maintaining of an open and trusting relationship with Gill. There were times, particularly in the early days, when she was very tense when visiting the clinic and aggression seemed very near the surface. It was useful to have the additional contact through CFRT as she was an enthusiastic fund-raiser. On her own admission she was very independent and did not readily ask for help, but she did, in fact, ask for assistance on the two occasions described above. She commented on the last occasion, "I just needed someone to talk to". It seemed all too easy for clashes to arise with professional staff, whether in the hospital or at school, and it seemed important to maintain a supportive relationship in a low-key manner, available when needed, keeping up an interest in the family's welfare, but not pushing help or advice which was not wanted. In the discussions about the school trip I deliberately questioned Duncan about his feelings and encouraged him to speak for himself, and I hoped that this might get the message across to Gill that he was growing up and had opinions worthy of exploration and consideration. She did accept a comment from me in that context which had made her very angry when suggested by the school doctor, that is, that other children might be upset by Duncan's expectoration. Although I was unable to achieve the desired outcome on that occasion, Gill seemed to derive some comfort from my expression of depression and frustration after the school visit, saying, "I thought it was just me".

The twist to the tale is that at the beginning of 1989, when sweat tests were repeated, Shona was pronounced clear, as expected. Apparently out of the blue, Duncan's sweat test was also normal and they were told at the clinic that he did not have CF. I had advance warning of this happening and wondered how Gill would react, knowing that she normally operated 'on a short fuse'. She was dumbfounded, but kept laughing in incredulous relief between her questions. That relief was not replaced by anger; she was able to accept the reality of diagnostic difficulty, but she was concerned about the effect it would have on Duncan's confidence in the medical profession and about his current health status. Duncan was initially extremely angry; the focus he was able to express was that now Shona would never have to come to the clinic and he still had to come as he had asthma. A few days later when I visited at home he said that he felt better about it. His mother had said to him later on the day they were given the news, "Well if you've got asthma you can get treatment for it, but if it's CF there's no cure for it, you'd die of it". Duncan added, "So she said, 'Will we go in here and have a three course meal for a celebration?' - so we did, and I felt better after that".

I asked him if he had ever realised how serious CF was, or could be. He said, "Well I did and I didn't". He could not get the words together and Gill took over:

I think he didn't think about it. I don't think anyone can in that situation, you just can't think about it or you couldn't get on with day-to-day life. That'd be the first way to a nervous breakdown.

Hugh was quietly relieved:

Well - delighted that he doesn't have CF - but - there's still something, so I suppose there's still some worry. I'm sorry for the kids that do have it. We'll still be involved, raising money for research... There's the feeling - we haven't pushed him at school, thinking if he got to 16 or 17 - beyond that it's a bonus - so we thought we'd rather school was as enjoyable as possible. Now we'll be pushing him for the next two years. Fortunately he's quite bright, and he's interested in computers.

The comment on his being "quite bright" was an interesting turn-round suggesting a change in perception, as both parents had given the impression during the life history interviews of regarding Duncan as not very bright, although this may have been more related to a lack of application than a lack of innate ability.

The next hospital appointment was something of a let-down as all the necessary information was not to hand and a comprehensive review could not be made. The doctor promised to follow it up, which he did, and hospital admission was arranged so that full investigation of Duncan's health problem could be undertaken. I gave Duncan a lift home in the car and tried to elicit how he felt about the situation. He agreed first of all that he was fed up with it all, because he could not understand a word the doctor was saying, nor what his mother was saying to the doctor. I said that I thought his mother felt that it had affected him, because he knew he had CF and that would mean he would not have an adult life, so he had not worked much at school, and now he could look forward to a normal life. He said that was not right as far as he was concerned, he knew that he had CF, he did the things he had to do, like take his enzymes at lunch-time, but apart from that he did not think about it at all, just got on with the tasks to be done. He felt that he had got it in balance, doing what he had to do about it, but not letting it take over his life. Having established how he dealt with having CF, I tried to get at how he was now dealing with not having it. He found that hard, but did make some comment about hoping he would not find there had been something he should have been doing and it was too late to do anything about it. He thought though that if he did not have to make frequent trips to hospital any more, he would maybe be able to forget about it after a couple of years or so. There had been mention at the clinic of "nasty infections" and other diseases which may have raised fears that something sinister might yet be found.

113

Matters worsened when one consultant insisted that Duncan did have "a form of CF" and it became clear that, if CF was to be abandoned as a diagnosis, an alternative would have to be found, since Duncan did have a chronic lung problem of some kind. When Gill told me about the interview she was very angry, yet had the humour to say, "If you haven't finished your thesis, I don't know how you'll put this bit in". The uncertainty was very hard to live with. Gill said in hurt bewilderment, "Where do we go from here?". Duncan decided that the consultant was right, and that he did have CF, and expressed his anger against the doctors who were saying otherwise. While confusion continued he began to refuse to do his physiotherapy and to use his inhalers; Gill recognised this as teen-age rebellion but said:

Why, if he insists he's got CF, is he not doing his physio? He seems to want to have it, because then he'll be namby-pambied and everyone'll be sorry for him, yet he won't take the treatment for it.

Since in recent months Duncan had used me as confidante on more than one occasion, I offered to call in and have a chat with him but Gill felt that he was at such an awkward stage that it would not matter who spoke to him, he would still be difficult. I offered to lend her a book on adolescence, which she accepted. The lengthy period of uncertainty has been extremely difficult and until an alternative diagnosis can be confirmed the family is suspended, uncertain how to face the future.

The Armstrong family

My first visit to this family was as a follow-up to a clinic visit at which it appeared that Mrs Armstrong was anticipating some difficulty in explaining her son's condition to school staff. Figure 10 provides a summary of the family structure.

Chris was 29 when we met in August 1983, Robert who had CF was five and Peter was two and a half. Her husband Jack worked as a welder and had recently been on unpaid sick leave following surgery on his spine, as well as having an eight-month period of redundancy. Chris had worked in an office before the birth of her first child; she said that she was now enjoying motherhood. She worked two evenings a week in her parents' pub. The family lived in a three-apartment top flat. The boys slept in a box-room with bunk beds. They had hoped to move to a house with a garden but financial setbacks had postponed this.

Because Robert had no symptoms of CF, the pre-diagnostic stage was brief and atypical.

Pre-diagnostic stage

The first suggestion of there being a problem came when Chris took Robert to the clinic for a routine check-up. The doctor asked her if she thought his chest protruded a little. She said:

> I didn't, but then as soon as I got him home I had him lying down and sitting up, because as soon as someone says something like that to you, you immediately think "Well if they thought that, it must".

The doctor said there was nothing to worry about, but she should mention it to her GP when she next saw him. She did so two weeks later because she was pregnant by then with Peter. She remembered that there was a locum there as well as the older doctor; the locum did not think there was anything wrong with him, "he said everybody's chest's different", but the older doctor said that, just to put her mind at rest, he would send Robert to see a professor at the Children's Hospital. This was done and there were blood tests and an X-ray, "and all sorts of examinations", then a sweat test:

> I got the result, and the result said, nothing to worry about, but his sweat test is abnormally high. But I didn't know what they were doing the sweat test for. The people that were doing it said they were collecting sweat from his body, but I was still anxious to know why they were collecting sweat from his body, but at that time they didn't tell me, or couldn't tell me.... After the second sweat test, they still didn't tell me what it was for until they actually

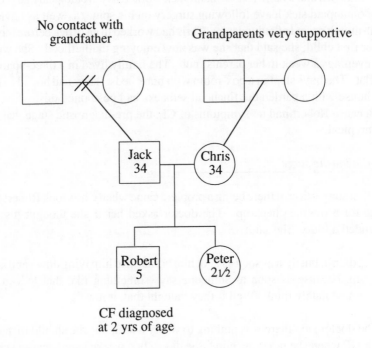

No contact with
grandfather

Grandparents very supportive

Jack
34

Chris
34

Robert
5

Peter
2½

CF diagnosed
at 2 yrs of age

Figure 10
The Armstrong family genogram: 1983

sent for me, and they said they thought he had cystic fibrosis.

Confrontational stage

Chris looked back on that period as being "quite horrendous":

> Yes, well, in early pregnancy it was very hard because well your emotions are upside down anyway, then somebody telling you that you've got a baby that's abnormal and that's not going to live, and he seems perfectly healthy to you. But that was very hard to believe ... So em ... I found that it spoiled my pregnancy as well, for the next few months, worrying if the baby was going to have it as well. I couldn't accept it, as Robert having CF because he'd been such a well child and it was really, really upsetting. And it was even more upsetting when I found out what it was.

When she was told that the baby would be tested after birth she picked up the idea that the baby would be taken away from her right after the birth. The baby was born "fine and healthy". Chris commented on how distressing it had been to have her baby taken away after every feed for a blood test and to hear him crying while they were taking blood from him. If any explanation was given it was not understood:

> C   I didn't really know what that was ... So he had a sweat test when he was about six weeks old and they found out that his sweat test was OK and he was fine. But they said they'd keep an eye on Peter anyway when I was at the hospital with Robert.

> DW Did that leave you with a question, whether Peter was really alright?

> C   Well what happened when Peter did have the sweat test I 'phoned up one of the doctors and she thought the sweat test was abnormal, so that was frightening again and very upsetting. But then again when I actually saw the doctor it was a different doctor and he said there was nothing wrong with Peter's sweat, he was OK.

Jack, Chris's husband, seems to have felt much the same as Chris did, he too having no previous knowledge of CF. Robert remained well and his parents learned to give him physiotherapy twice a day and to encourage him to take plenty of exercise. They were told just to keep an eye on his bowel movements. On my second home visit Chris recalled that it was when the home visiting nurse was in that the full impact of CF was realised. As the nurse was explaining it, Chris said, "You make it sound like a dreaded killer disease", "Well it is", came the reply.

117

The genetic aspects of CF added to the stress of that period. Chris felt that she had been more affected by this than her husband:

> You begin to blame yourself ... It took such a long time to come to terms that it really wasn't my fault after all.

Her parents were also upset. It was three or four years before she was able to tell her brothers about it:

> ... they couldn't believe it either, because they thought he was so well and so healthy, and then they were concerned themselves. Because one brother already had two children but the others were just about to start a family. They had a baby and they tested him and he was OK.

Chris reckoned that it was fully a year before she and her husband came to terms with the diagnosis. She felt that they moved through this stage at very much the same pace. They could speak about it together, but at that time Chris had not been able to tell any of her family, apart from her parents.

Long-term adaptive stage

Robert continued to keep well, and every clinic visit showed him to be above average height and to be gaining weight steadily. Chris commented that the health visitors who called in during his pre-school years had little knowledge of CF. She questioned me about my nursing background and my involvement with CF, and seemed interested, and perhaps relieved, to hear that I had nursed a number of children with CF. She accepted that the doctors could not predict the course of the illness for each individual and that she therefore did not know how severely Robert would be affected in later years. She and Jack went together to the CFRT meetings and she felt that her knowledge of the disease was increasing. She told me on three separate occasions of the time she was at the clinic with Robert and was querying how it was that Robert was not showing any of the symptoms of CF. The consultant said, "Just wait till he's a bit older, and he will have". She said that hurt her deeply and she was determined to prove him wrong if she could.

When he was about six Robert "took a bad turn" and was taken straight up to the hospital. He was admitted and kept in for about five days. It was said then that he was having an asthmatic attack, and the doctors suggested that he was asthmatic and perhaps did not have CF at all. In December 1984, when we met at a CFRT meeting, Chris said that the sweat tests remainded borderline. She seemed then to be accepting the rather uncertain situation and one month later, during a home visit, she said, "I know there's something wrong with his chest, whether it's CF or not". We agreed that there were many degrees of severity of CF. Two years on, the doctor at the clinic was able to convince her that there was no need for a further sweat test and the monthly visits were discontinued. Even then Chris was not quite sure that he was clear; she had met a girl at the clinic who was in her twenties and she said that she only started coughing when she was 13 years old. In 1988 Robert was still well and I asked, "Do you believe it now?". The reply was:

> Well, yes ... there'll always be a question there. But he's a fine healthy boy
> - but I'll take extra care of him.

During the life history interview in early 1989 she said about the withdrawal of the diagnosis:

> Then I found that as hard to believe as when they said that he did have CF, after attending the hospital all those years ... But they couldn't say one hundred percent that he's OK, just as certain as they can be in medicine.

Jack's reactions again mirrored her own. Her parents were delighted. They were sad that he has asthma, but thought that it was easier to live with asthma than it was with CF:

DW   Do you feel that?

C   Oh yes, with CF you don't know if they're going to live, but I find - I can accept it more now that he doesn't have CF. It's easier now and I've got a good idea when he's going to have an asthma attack and I try to prevent it now ... We keep him very active, he swims a lot and he runs and he plays football and he's very sporty.

DW   Is there any anger around?

C   No, I don't feel angry. It was really upsetting at the time, but I don't feel angry about it. Otherwise I might not have known much about CF at all, even as yet. You hear more about it now.

DW   Mmhm, also you take it in more.

C   That's right, I'm much more involved with it now. So no, I'm not angry.

DW   And you don't feel you just want to cut off from it?

C   No, no ... No ... I'm really quite interested in it now.

DW   Mmhm. What about decisions about family, did it influence your decisions?

C   Yes, well when Robert was diagnosed I was advised not to have any more children. At that time I was already pregnant and after that they advised me not to have any more, which, em, well I took their advice but I would probably have liked more, well another one anyway, but em, I don't feel angry about that either, not now anyway. But I mean that decision was made for me and I just decided to take the advice the doctors had given but I don't feel upset about it now.

In spite of her protestations, I had the distinct impression from Chris's facial expression and tone of voice that this was quite an upsetting area. I did not probe further at the time, but made reference later to her even temperament. She agreed but said that her problem when she was upset was eating. She found it hard to stop eating once she started, and had to be very careful to stop herself from becoming overweight. Her husband had the same kind of problem.

Robert had never asked many questions about his illness. He developed something of a phobia about needles, which dated back to an occasion when he was three and was held down to have a venepuncture. He described it as "having a screwdriver put in my arm to take the blood out". His anxieties seemed to relate directly to blood tests at the hospital rather than the outcome of his illness. He now knew that he did not have CF because he no longer attended the hospital, but took an interest in the fund-raising activities of the CFRT, in which his mother was involved.

Peter had enjoyed the hospital visits, playing with the toys and going into all the different rooms. He knew about CF and was interested in the fund-raising activities also, but Chris doubted if he really knew what CF was and felt he was not too worried about it.

When asked what had helped her to come to terms with CF and the 'Why us?' questions, she said:

Well we didn't really have any feelings of 'Why us?', we just accepted that if the doctor said he had it, then he had it, and we just had to live with it, and cope with it, and take it day by day. We just used to hope and pray that they were wrong ... Well I thought personally, well if there's any way that I can care for him, that'll make him not to have it, well he won't have it . That helped ... I realise now though that if he had actually had CF, no matter how much you care and nurse for them, it's genetic and it's there - it will progress - but I just prayed that he wouldn't have it, that they'd made a mistake and dealt with it that way.

Crisis points and the time factor

The investigations and then the diagnosis of CF formulated the initial hazardous event. In view of how well Robert had been, it seemed quite possible that there would be no such events. Figure 11, however, represents the crises identified by Chris.

Chest infections The chest infections came readily to her mind when I asked, "Is there any time, since diagnosis, that sticks out in your mind as a bit of a crisis time, or particularly difficult?", Chris said:

> He has had a couple of chest infections, em, I always remember them, because of being in the position that they said he had CF ...

The hospital admission was seen as a crisis, as might be expected, but it was made more stressful by the fact that Robert "hated hospitals so much" because of his fear of blood tests. Chris remembered that he was distraught every time they took blood from him.

Withdrawal of the diagnosis of CF While the news that Robert did not have CF was more than welcome, the transition back to normality from the acceptance of being a family with a health problem was not easy, as has been indicated.

Time

Chris referred to the time it took for her and her husband to come to terms with Robert's diagnosis. That was about a year and, ironically, it was more like two years before she was convinced that the diagnosis had been incorrect. The threat of time was seen in her acceptance that Robert's prognosis could not be predicted and they would just have to wait to see how things went for him - underlined painfully by the doctor's comment that the symptoms would come. Part of the process of acceptance was the resolve to "take it day by day". Then there was the element of hope. When she was talking about Robert's asthma, Chris said, "Hopefully every seven years or so, they say ... hopefully we'll get rid of that as well".

121

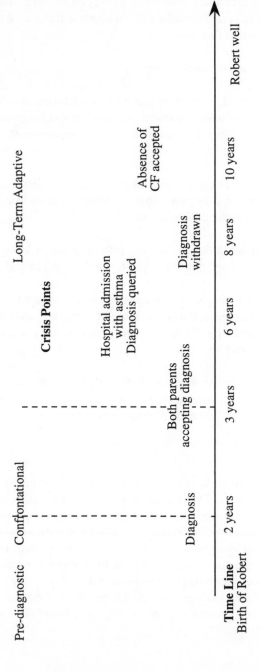

Figure 11

Stages of the family's experience in adapting to illness related to time and to crisis points

Basic and developmental tasks: family interaction

It is difficult to make a detailed assessment of this family's achievement of these tasks as I had so little contact with family members apart from the mother. The impression is of a close-knit family with the stress of cystic fibrosis failing to disrupt harmonious relationships. There is no evidence that family life was deleteriously affected by the experience of CF, although it undoutedly imposed serious stress and indeed influenced the limitation of family size. It seemed, however, that the family was able to integrate the uncomfortable knowledge into its functioning and make it work positively. The need for exercise for Robert drew the whole family closer as they went swimming and walking together. There seemed to be a fairly impermeable family boundary, in that for some years only the maternal grandparents were told of the diagnosis. Help from sources outside the family were however accepted, for example, the home visiting nurse and contact with other CF parents through the CFRT. The continuing trust in the medical profession is notable, and perhaps reflects a mature ability to tolerate the ambiguity of being dependent on medical knowledge and expertise while accepting that it is fallible. It also suggests socialisation into the belief that 'doctors know best', firmly held in spite of evidence to the contrary.

Nursing support

My input in this case was modified to meet a situation in which the initial information had been given and received, and the child was healthy in spite of the grave diagnosis. The offer of support in informing school staff about CF was not required as Chris dealt with this herself, and was relieved to find that the headmistress already had a considerable knowledge of CF. Frequent home visiting was clearly not necessary as the family was managing the treatment requirements and the mother seemed to be handling the stress of the grim prognosis well. There were informal contacts through the CFRT, however, and a friendly relationship developed easily in which anxieties could be shared. Often these related more to family matters such as Jack's job, the threat and reality of redundancy, the mortgage for the new home, a fatal accident to a child in the street, than to the daily demands of CF. I was able to support Chris's need to limit to some degree her involvement with CFRT fundraising activities as there were at times demands which were unreasonable for someone with two young children and a husband to consider. I offered some advice with regard to Robert's fear of injections and with regard to contacting her GP on a later occasion when Robert was "coughing terribly". Chris seemed reticent about making this contact, possibly feeling less justified in voicing her anxiety since the grave diagnosis no longer applied. As has been indicated, the uncertainties about the diagnosis were discussed and the gradual acceptance was observed.

The Dean family

Donald and Mary Dean were in their mid-30's when we met; Lesley was ten and Stephen, who had cystic fibrosis, was eight. The family lived in a three-bedroomed owner-occupied house in an attractive estate on the edge of Edinburgh. The house was always immaculate and the garden was usually kept neat and tidy. Family structure is shown in Figure 12.

In examining the experience of this family the early stages were more difficult to define because of the fact that the first child, Anne, died of cystic fibrosis aged 23 months. In relation to this brief life the pre-diagnostic and confrontational stages are clear, but as the time span from diagnosis to death was only six months, the long-term adaptive stage and the terminal stage merge together, leaving a young couple in their early twenties devastated by their loss.

Since this occurrence would be bound to impinge on later parenting experience, the relevant data obtained during the life history interview in which both parents participated are presented first, setting the scene for subsequent events in the life of the family.

Pre-diagnostic stage

Mary felt from the time Anne was nine months old that there was something wrong; she had a troublesome cough and had alternate diarrhoea and constipation. Her own mother felt that there was something wrong but did not want to worry Mary. Donald's mother was reassuring, saying that Donald too had problems with his bowels as a baby. By the time Anne was one year old, Mary was convinced there was a problem as the baby was not gaining weight. Of this stage she said:

> I just felt I was banging my head against a brick wall because they'd say, 'A winter baby, bound to be chesty', or 'That's teeth', or all the excuses of the day. You felt you were a neurotic Mum.

Donald acknowledged that Mary was the first to be worried; "You never really visualised there's something seriously wrong". They changed their general practitioner three times during this period and, even then, when Anne was 17 months old and really ill, Mary had difficulty in convincing the doctor that it was anything serious. She was, however, given an appointment to see a consultant, who admitted Anne from the clinic. The baby was treated for severe pneumonia and a week later the diagnosis of cystic fibrosis was made.

124

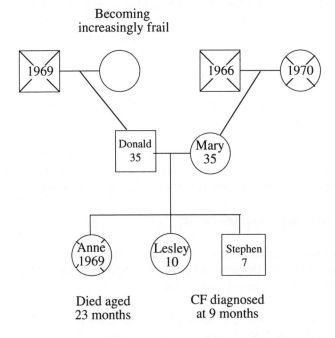

Figure 12
The Dean family genogram: 1983

They were both stunned by the news and it seemed that much of what was said was not comprehended. Mary said:

> It didn't really register, although he told us what it was, I never thought she could die of it ... I always remembered about a fortnight before she died, he called us in and told us. He maybe just didn't want to put us through all that at the time. We were so young, maybe he thought it was too much for us to take in at one time.

It was the genetic nature of the illness that most upset Donald. He expressed his reactions vividly:

> I really felt as if you were going about with two horns growing out of your head, there was a physical abnormality about you, and even talking to the family, you felt as if they knew there was something wrong wi' you.

Mary admitted to a sense of guilt:

> ... obviously you feel it's your fault that the baby's like that, I felt guilty, but I didn't feel like Donald did, like I was going about with this big sign on my head, saying, 'I've got faulty genes'.

She felt frustrated because nobody she spoke to knew anything about cystic fibrosis; they'd say, "What's that, is that like fibrositis?".
The stress of the situation had an adverse effect on the marriage. Mary said:

> I just couldnae stand it. He was getting violent. I thought, 'I just cannae cope wi' this'. He just seemed to fly off the handle - not beat me up, but you know, maybe give me a slap across the face, you know, for stupid wee things. I thought, 'This is going to land up me being a battered wife' kind o' thing.

Donald agreed, "It was really terrible". Mary told Donald's mother about it, and she came up to the house with his father and they spoke to him. "Whatever they said", Mary commented, "it worked".
Donald tried to explain how he had felt at the time:

> I was 22, roughly, and I felt as though I was in the prime of my life, and basically you'd been hit below the belt by this - how could you say - brand

126

on you. As Mary said, I'd come in from my work, where everyone's jolly, no problems, and I'd come back into the house, and Mary'd be late back from the shops and was making the meal and it was just an excuse to fly off the handle.

He recalled his parents had said to him:

It's the best friend you're ever going to have ... and basically you've got to share everything together and a burden shared is a burden halved.

He thought more about it, and realised Mary's mother was also unwell at the time and that Mary had more than enough to do. He said:

... in that respect it bonded us together. But it might not have worked, if people hadn't had - like I say - my parents.

There could only have been a brief period of adaptation before Anne died. Nothing was said directly about the pain of that experience, but there was passing reference to it later when describing the stress of illness in their second child. A factor which greatly compounded the grief of losing Anne was the advice they were given that they should have no more children. To Mary:

It was like the end of the world when he said that, I was absolutely devastated at the thought of no being able to have any more kids.

There was no specific advice about sterilisation; adoption was mentioned and the consultant told them to keep in touch with him and that if he could help in any way he would.

Donald's father was again a source of strength in helping his son to cope with his grieving. Donald said:

He was trying to give some support and compassion for the days to come, he was saying 'It's maybe a blessing that she didn't live longer, it'd have been harder for you'. It was comforting at the time, you know, because he said, 'Nobody can take the memory away, nobody's got that but you'. That stayed me in great stead for the days to come.

Sadly, Donald's father and Mary's mother both died in the year following the death of Anne. The young couple felt bitter and bewildered but attempted to re-organise their lives:

We wanted our lives back into a normality if you can say that, after all this with Anne, and we moved house. It was more harrowing for Mary than it was for me ... because she was in the house most of the day wi' Anne, you know ... I had the escapism, to go away to my work in the morning ... And quite rightly we decided to move, and we moved. And again, when we moved house, friends gave us support and it was quite good, it was like starting our marriage again ...

Mary commented:

You needed it, something like that, you didnae have time to sit and think and brood about things because there was that much to do in the house, that had to be done.

Donald continued:

We had to replumb it, rewire it and redecorate it. It took quite a long time. And that, eh, really bonded our marriage, eh, in that respect, then Lesley came along, and that was great.

The pregnancy occurred just after the couple had been accepted as adoptive parents. The genetic implications cast a shadow over what would otherwise have been a joyous event. Mary said, "That was horrendous as well, with one saying it should be aborted ...". They confided in the consultant, who advised terminating the pregnancy. They accepted that he was looking at it from more experience of the disease than they were, with just the six months of Anne's illness behind them, and that he had been trying to spare them suffering. When he saw that they wanted to go on with the pregnancy he referred them to an obstetrician and they had three consultations before they made their final decision. Mary remembered:

He just listened. But when we finally made the decision, he said, "I'm glad you've made that decision, because in the frame of mind you're in, if you had the baby aborted it'd have a drastic effect, even worse than if you had the baby and lost it". So he was in agreement with us carrying on with the pregnancy.

Donald commented:

To be honest, I left the major decision to Mary. I said I'd willingly go along wi' her decision, which was putting an untold burden on Mary's decision-making ... Possibly I was more for going through with the pregnancy, to be

128

honest, the reason for going in for the adoption was that everything was for a family, if you see what I mean.

They agreed that their own tragedy and their desire to found a family combined to cause a considerable bitterness, particularly when they felt that others around them were casual about their children's welfare. Mary was particularly upset by her sister who told her when she was pregnant that she should have "it" aborted:

> I used to think, 'Look at her, she's caused that much trouble to my mother, and has these two children - perfectly healthy - that she didn't want, that she'll palm off onto anyone that'll have them, and here was me, desperately wanting a child, and she's telling me to get rid of the one I'm carrying'. That still sticks in my throat.

Following Lesley's birth, Mary was advised to see a paediatrician and she chose to go back to the original consultant since he knew the past history:

> I'd been through such a harrowing experience, I thought I don't want to go and have to go through the whole thing, and get upset - it's emotional enough when you've just had a baby.

Nevertheless, she was a bit nervous about going back to the consultant whose advice regarding abortion had not been accepted. Donald had reassured her on this point, "And it couldn't really have worked out any better for us; it's been sort of a lifetime relationship".

Lesley was a contented baby who fed and slept well; although there was a vague anxiety at the back of Mary's mind, predominantly both parents were just delighted with their daughter. When she was three months old she took bronchitis quite badly and when Mary telephoned the hospital she was told to bring her to the clinic that day. She was admitted and nursed in a croupette. Mary said:

> That was really ... when I saw her in the croupette, it was just like Anne, it brought it all back.

Donald interjected:

> I used to have nightmares about it ... seeing her in the croupette ... I hated it ... when I saw Lesley in it, I thought, 'That's it, she's got it, she's going to die as well ...

Their fears were not realised. Lesley responded very quickly to treatment, they were assured that she did not have CF and thereafter she "really blossomed as a baby".The family moved house again, by which time Mary was pregnant with Stephen. I asked if they had the same kind of agonizing over whether to have him or not, the way they did with Lesley. Mary explained:

> With Lesley it was a different situation because we'd just lost a child and desperately wanted another one, it was just a different situation altogether. Personally, for me, I wanted to take the chance, whether or not she had CF I just wanted another child. I wasnae caring if it had two heads, I mean that was the way I looked at it. But it was different when I was deciding about Stephen, because Lesley was definitely healthy. 'It couldnae happen ... she's fine'.

The stages of adaptation through which the family passed in relation to Stephen's illnes can now be considered.

Pre-diagnostic stage

Stephen was the heaviest of the three babies when he was born and seemed healthy; he fed well and put on weight. Because of the family history he had a stool test at birth which was normal, but not thought to be very reliable. He had a sweat test at three months, which was normal and another at seven months, which was borderline. The consultant put him on pancreatic enzymes and physiotherapy when he was three months of age, saying that it was purely precautionary and would do no harm if he did not have CF. Looking back, they realised that the consultant must have made his diagnosis earlier but it was not confirmed by a positive sweat test until Stephen was nine months old. Because he seemed healthy, put on weight and had fairly normal stools, his parents did not anticipate the diagnosis.

Confrontational stage

When the bad news was given at the clinic, Mary was shocked, the more so because she had been told over the telephone that the third sweat test was normal. She concluded that the registrar must have been looking at the second result but she wondered how anyone could make such a mistake. She had been elated, thinking that he did not have CF:

> ... honestly, you could have knocked me down with a feather when Dr A said 'I'm sorry' ... because I wasn't worried because he was that healthy looking.

130

Donald said:

> After that initial period, you were still shocked, but it wasn't such a traumatic shock as Anne because he wasn't ill. He was well. Anne was ill when she was diagnosed and that was horrific. But Stephen was well and healthy and diagnosed.

Since the consultant had said that there were different severities of CF and because Stephen was so healthy, Mary concluded:

> I had it in my mind, well, he's just got it very mild. He's one of these kids that would go unnoticed. But it wasn't, it was just because he'd been treated early.

Donald agreed:

> Well I knew the disease was a progressive disease ... but it was comforting from the point of view that Stephen was well, and had been diagnosed, so that was a comfort and what I did say, if I remember, was, 'Well, he's diagnosed, it was nearly five years since Anne's death, and a lot's been happening in that five years, bythe time another five years comes, there'll be a lot more happening. They'll easily have a better treatment.

It seems that because of their earlier experience the family was able to progress fairly rapidly to the long-term adaptive stage, which they were in when I first had contact with them. This stage has many facets and repeated illnesses and spells in hospital placed a considerable strain on the family's adaptive strengths. The following is a synthesis of data from field notes and from the life history interviews.

Long-term adaptive stage: the affected child

Following the diagnosis, Stephen had no real health problems until he was three years of age and when he was admitted to hospital at four years, the parents were told that he had pseuodomonas in his sputum; he was in and out of hospital every three to four months during the following year. The year before our meeting had been a relatively good one and a recent illness had been treated at home, with district nurses coming in to give intramuscular antibiotics.

At eight years of age, Stephen was active and enjoyed football and disco dancing, although he tired fairly quickly. He tended to try to prove himself in this area and a recent school report had said that he took a very active part in physical education classes. He was an intelligent child and, although he did not enjoy school, he coped fairly easily with it. He had a quick tongue and a lively sense of humour. He could be very irritable at times with his family, particularly with his mother, but was also very affectionate. He became a firm favourite with hospital staff, who enjoyed his fun and teasing, although one or two members of staff found his cheekiness difficult to manage.

In making the initial health assessment I learned that Stephen normally ate well, but he became anorexic whenever he was unwell. His mother reckoned that this, along with becoming irritable and complaining of sore legs, was the first sign that he was becoming ill. His stools were mostly normal, two times per day; sometimes they were 'porridgy' looking and occasionally he would have four or five stools in a day. When they were loose at these times they were smelly and Stephen found this embarrassing at school. He coughed a lot and expectorated which also caused some problems at school. One classmate protested, 'You're poisoning the ground'. Stephen was very interested in physiotherapy and listened to the explanations he was given. He had taught a neighbour the technique and also kept his aunt right when he stayed with her overnight. He was able to manage his own personal hygiene but his parents tended to help him more than usual because he took so long about it, particularly in the mornings.

Mary coped with the demands of the treatment regime with cheerfulness and fortitude, but both parents admitted that when Stephen became ill they became irritable and 'narky' with each other. After one particularly stressful episode Mary felt that she was having to cope with everything and that it was too much. They came to an agreement that Donald would take over the evening physiotherapy. On more than one occasion she said, "The only rows in this house are about Stephen and his physio". The difficulties, however, were not removed by this strategy as Stephen sometimes reported to his mother that Donald had not been doing the physiotherapy properly - "He's looking out the window and not looking at what he's doing". This upset Mary who would then let fly at Donald with a comment like, "It's his life that's at stake - it's up to you". Having sparked off the row, Stephen would sit back and watch television while his parents argued.

Such overtly manipulative behaviour was not frequently evidenced. It was, however, Mary who bore the brunt of Stephen's anger and frustration when he was unwell. During one of his spells in hospital he was being so cheeky that Mary slapped him, then had to leave because she was so upset. He had been a bit quiet for a day or two but soon regained his usual sparkle, and it did curb his cheekiness for a time. Mary admitted that she worried about him getting wet and restricted his outdoor activity accordingly. She usually drove him to school by car, although it was within fairly easy walking distance. She also tended to discourage swimming.

In hospital it was noticed that when he was unwell he became irritable and

132

fussed over his meals and physiotherapy. He could be very angry with his great friend, the play leader, although she noted too in her diary that he gave his mother a hard time when he was feeling low. In earlier days his anger could be expressed by bombing the castle he had made, but as time went on he became more philosophical about having to be in hospital.

Stephen became aware that he had an illness when the district nurses were coming in and giving him injections. He remembered:

> S   I was coughing all the time and wondering what it was, and my Mum said, 'You've got gunge in your lungs', and I says, 'What's that?'. And she said, 'It's just green stuff, germs and that in your chest, that's how you're getting the jags, and you're getting better'. So then I realised, that I kept getting this every now and then, and the nurse coming in and giving me jags, so it sort of clicked, 'poison in my system'. So I used to take tablets with my meals as well, and I wondered why I was gettin' it an' no-one else was, capsules spread all over my dinner and it made my dinner all runny an' horrible. So one day I decided, 'I'm not wantin' that, my sister's no gettin' it, so I climbed down' one morning and took my capsules ... and put them in the washing machine, in the soap powder bit, and my Mum put the machine on and the nappies an' everything came out all green. So I got a row for that.

> DW   That was you trying to get rid of them, was it?

> S   Aye. That was when I first knew about it.

He reckoned he was two or three at that time, then, when he was four, he was admitted to hospital:

> I didnae really like it much, started getting drips and that, instead of getting it in my bottom ... an' I started saying, 'This is more than a chest infection' ... I cannae really remember my Mum ever telling me I had cystic fibrosis, I just sortae went along wi' it, an' found out about it myself.

He demonstrated his skills in communication at an early age:

> S   I knew I had something, but I asked my Mum, 'What's it called again?'. She says, 'What?'. 'My thingy that I've got'. She says, 'Cystic fibrosis'. But she never sat me down and told me I'd got it, I found out for myself.

DW   Would you have liked her to sit you down and tell you?

S   Naw, it was better she done it the way she done it.

Long-term adaptive stage: the parents

Mary's health and well-being tended to reflect Stephen's wellness and illness. At one point she went to her general practitioner because she was feeling so tired and unwell; he did not give her a prescription, saying, "You won't be better till Stephen's better". He was right. She admitted to being a "comfort eater" and had considerable problems keeping her weight down. A preoccupation with dieting perhaps helped to deflect some of her attention and anxiety from Stephen. She had given up working during one of Stephen's spells in hospital, but later was pleased to be able to take a part-time job working two or three nights a week in a home for the elderly. Although this was tiring, she appreciated the flexibility it gave her to cope with hospital appointments and in-patient stays.

Donald worked as a maintenance engineer, which he found rather boring, but he maintained other interests such as Boys' Brigade and sport. He had a good relationship with Stephen and took him out frequently. He encouraged Stephen's interest in football but, as time went on, he appreciated that his son was not able to keep up with the other boys. If Stephen showed signs of self-pity he would jolly him out of it, and if he was frustrated and tense he would suggest a bicycle ride and the two might go off together. He twice mentioned the difficulty in coping with the contrasting experience of work and home life. There was a continuing pressure in the feeling that workmates "don't realise what you've got to go through in your daily life". One of the things he found hardest to bear was the inability of friends and family to accept that there was something wrong with Stephen. He felt that when he and Mary "went into action" whenever Stephen developed a cold, the family thought they were being over-protective. Even though they had explained the illness and tried to help the family to understand, they found that people still said things like, "Will he no grow out o' it?".

Their experience of death and illness initially shattered their faith and left them bitter. Mary admitted that she hated God for several years and had a fear of having Lesley baptised, "... it was ridiculous, but I felt that if I had her christened, God would take her away". Donald was just "switched off". Over the past five years or so their attitudes had changed and during the interview Donald identified faith in God as his principal support:

> I mean he's become approachable, every day, no just Sunday. In that respect, you can say your friends and your family ... it's humanistic support and comfort, knowing that they'll help you with the physical effort, they're

134

no lightening your burden in any way, because your looking for spiritual support. It only lightens the task, it's never taking the burden and being free ... I wonder if CF was given to bring us back, because we'd wandered, to bring us back to test our faith. It's a hard test to go through, if you didnae have that faith, you'd be really cracking up ... This faith, and power and prayer, that's a great help to me.

Mary named friends and family as her chief support, and spoke also of the strength she gained from the doctors and nurses at the hospital:

... although they're not personal friends, you've been going there for so long and you know everyone's rooting for you.

She no longer rejected God but admitted that she still asked "Why?". There were times when the meaning of it all seemed clear, other times - usually when Stephen was unwell - when she felt that she was being put to the test again:

Sometimes I feel as if I'm completely in God's hands. My life's mapped out, this has been His way.

Mary felt that Stephen put it all in perspective for her. He had said that this was what God was waiting for, for this chance of a transplant to come:

He can't make him well, he's got too much to mend. Stephen said, the first time we took him to a healing service, 'I know I'll no be healed right away, because I've had it since I was born, it'd take too long to reverse the situation'. So a new heart and lungs is the best way of repairing his abnormalities.

She had an experience in prayer:

It was like somebody putting arms around me and saying 'Everything'll be fine. I know you worry, but it'll all come alright'.

Long-term adaptive stage: the healthy sibling

Lesley, at ten years of age, was slightly plump and lacking in self-confidence. Her mother reckoned that she was jealous of all the attention Stephen was given. She would often say things like, "If he asked for it, he'd get it". She was slower than Stephen at school and he would correct her. She was less open about her feelings, although she was very kind hearted; Mary said she was the first to befriend a new

135

immigrant family who came to the neighbourhood.

The clearest indication of her feelings was recounted to me by Mary in 1987, the day after they had watched a television film together. The film had been about a brain-damaged child and the parents' fight for her recovery. The brother had been displaying anti-social behaviour and Lesley commented, "I know what's wrong with him, he's jealous of the attention his sister's getting". Later, when the son and his father were having an open and distressed talk about the problems, Lesley was crying. Mary felt that Lesley was moody at that time, although she was very good with Stephen and had taken him to town for the first time that weekend. Around that time, when the family was on an outing, Stephen injured his ankle and had to be taken to hospital. Lesley's frustrated reaction was, "Why does it always have to be him?".

During the life history interview it seemed that Lesley had no clear memory of finding out about Stephen having CF, although she remembered the incident of the enzymes in the washing machine. She remembered her mother having to change doctors:

> ... because she didn't get anywhere. She had to do the same with Anne, she wasn't getting anywhere with Anne either, till she got Dr A.

She had learned about Anne when she was about ten or eleven, when her mother told her. She could tell me that Anne would be eighteen if she had lived and said wistfully, "I just wisht I had a big sister, I'd have liked one".

Crisis points and the time factor

There have been many crises. During the life history interview Donald and Mary identified three "crisis points"; from my field notes I picked out two other occasions when the family's resources seemed stretched almost to breaking point. A crisis of a spiritual nature arose in the final weeks of the study. The hazardous event again lay in the diagnosis of CF. The time sequence of crisis points is illustrated in Figure 13.

Drug error The drug error occurred when arrangements had been made for the district nurses to give Stephen his antibiotics by intramuscular injection. It was Donald who drew attention to the dosage and the nurses discovered that a double dose had been given for four days. The drug had a known side-effect of causing deafness and the mistake caused intense anxiety for a time, to Stephen as well as his parents. Donald said:

136

Figure 13

Stages of the family's experience in adapting to illness related to time and to crisis points

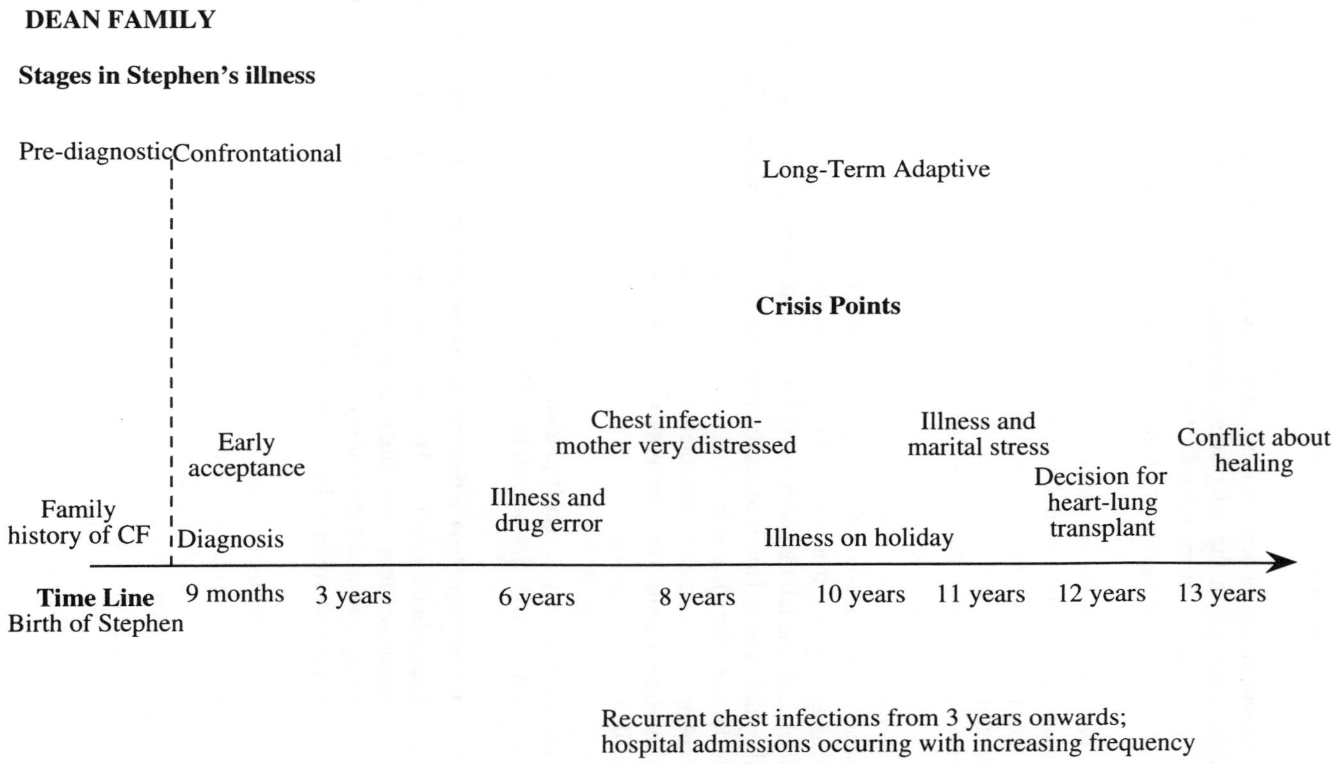

DEAN FAMILY

Stages in Stephen's illness

Pre-diagnostic｜Confrontational

Long-Term Adaptive

Crisis Points

Early
acceptance

｜Diagnosis

Chest infection-
mother very distressed

Illness and
drug error

Illness on holiday

Illness and
marital stress

Decision for
heart-lung
transplant

Conflict about
healing

Family history of CF								
Time Line Birth of Stephen	9 months	3 years	6 years	8 years	10 years	11 years	12 years	13 years

Recurrent chest infections from 3 years onwards;
hospital admissions occuring with increasing frequency

That was quite a horrific experience that, the aspect that it had been done, the strain it placed on myself, and the decision you had to come to at the end.

Donald telephoned the hospital and, having discussed it with the doctor on duty, insisted on the drug being stopped. The consultant had been at first incredulous about the mistake, but later was supportive and able to assure the parents that Stephen had not suffered any harmful effect.

Chest infection The episode of illness which I identified as a crisis point occurred a few months after my first contact with the family. Stephen's condition had been causing concern over the past few months; a second consultant had been called to give an opinion and Stephen had been admitted to hospital on two occasions. It was just before the second admission that Mary was so distressed that she admitted on the telephone that she had felt suicidal. When we discussed it later, it seemed to relate to the impact of Stephen's illness - he had fallen asleep in the school playground - and the fact that she had been unable to tell Donald how she was feeling. She was worried too by comparing Stephen with older children who looked ill and felt that, although he was considerably younger, he looked as ill as they did. She had felt it necessary to give up her work because of the time needed to be with Stephen in hospital. After she had spoken with Donald about her feelings she seemed better able to cope with the recurring stress. I noted at this time how openly the problems were discussed with me in front of the two children.

Illness on holiday A very frightening episode occurred some two years later. The family went to Wales on holiday. Donald commented:

> It really shook us to the extent how far Stephen would go to keep everyone happy in the family ... He would go along with Lesley, and walk along to shows an' that ... coming back he couldnae keep up with her, so he'd stop every now and then and say, 'Come and look at this', so although Lesley wasn't aware of it, he'd slow them down.

They decided to come home early and on their last day Stephen was "absolutely shattered", being carried on his father's back all day. They decided then to travel overnight to avoid the traffic and the heat of the day. They were all upset about it and debated whether they should go to hospital locally, but felt that a two or three week admission there should be avoided. They set off at midnight; Donald remembered, "So we got to Carlisle and it was really a bit frightening then". Mary explained, "He was white but everything else was blue, his lips and his ear and the end of his nose".

138

Donald stopped at a service station and telephoned the hospital ward; he told the staff how Stephen was and said that they should be there in two hours' time. He asked if there was a hospital in Carlisle that they should go to and the staff nurse said that if he was so bad they should really take him there and get him admitted. Donald was anxious, however, that Stephen would not respond to treatment in a strange hospital because he would not have the same faith in the staff. Mary said, "I was panicking, I just wanted to take him to Carlisle". Donald's view prevailed and they set off again, but ran into roadworks:

> Lesley, she was absolutely panicking. We were shouting, 'keep him up', and Lesley was that tired, she was shattered. And we were taking it out on her. She says, 'We'll have to stop' ... So I stopped the car and they were hanging out the side of the door and I says, 'Come on, get into the car, we're wasting valuable time here' ... I had to ... literally shove her in and got through the town and into the hosptial. They had everything ready ...

Mary said:

> It was terrible. I never thought he was going to make it to the hospital.

Lesley told the same story with little mention of herself, only that Stephen "looked awful". When I said that it must have been frightening, she said, "My Mum was most frightened". Stephen's comment to the play leader after that incident was, "Don't talk about it, I was very frightened". To another child he later said, "I nearly snuffed it at that time. I was nearly gone - but I didn't". That incident was thereafter viewed by the family and by the hospital staff as a low point in Stephen's illness 'career' which should be prevented from recurring if at all possible.

Illness and marital stress The fourth crisis point which I identified occurred some nine months later. Stephen was in hospital again and I telephoned the ward to ask how he was. The ward sister told me that Mary had just been sitting in the duty room weeping; Stephen was being very rude to her and she could take no more. She found it difficult to be hard on him in hospital because other parents may not understand. Stephen was not making much progress and was depressed. The ward staff were also finding difficulty with the question of discipline and consistency, and the sister had been intending to telephone me. She wanted to help but was at a loss to know how to do so. She also felt that there was increased tension within the marriage. I offered to visit later that evening and Mary accepted the offer.

Lesley was in, and seemed happy and cheerful, having just returned from a weekend away with her Bible class. She had been visiting Stephen in hospital and

139

commented on how 'narky' he was, and how he had called her 'Thickie' when they were playing a game together. Mary was looking pale and drawn and was arranging flowers sent by the church. Donald arrived a few minutes later; he had given Stephen his bath and hairwash, timed him running up the corridor, and left him bright and cheery.

When Lesley left us, they spoke for a few minutes of their concern about her school performance. She was given remedial work at school, but Mary felt that it should be more intensive. Lesley had burst into tears when it was mentioned, not wanting to be different from others at school.

In the ensuing discussion, the individual approach of each parent to handling Stephen was clearly portrayed. Donald reported a conversation a few days earlier, at home, in which Stephen was feeling low and moaning, "Why me?". Donald pointed out another child, who was paralysed, who had been in the news recently and said, "You're going to get better, there are plenty worse off than you". That tactic seemed to lift Stephen's mood and Donald implied that Mary was too sympathetic with him, that she "mothered" him too much, and perhaps should use what he called a "jokey" approach as well.

Mary recounted how she had gone in that day, taking his football album. She sat down and Stephen started looking for his stickers. "Where are my stickers?", he demanded. "I don't know - think where you had them last". "Help me then", he shouted. She reacted inwardly, "No, I won't help him". She felt deep down she wanted him to fight the illness, not to give in to it. He said, "Och, I'm fed up with this. I wish I wasnae here". She rounded on him then, "Do you think I've worked for you all these 11 years just for you to give up?". he took that in. I asked, "You feel he's seeing himself as ill?". "Yes", she said, "that's it".

This identified a problem of Stephen seeing himself as ill and dependent, and his parents' determination not to let that get a hold. I suggested that from Stephen's point of view the way they were dealing with his behaviour was probably about right; he felt safe to let out his anger and frustration at his mother, which was preferable to his turning in on himself and becoming withdrawn and depressed. He could then relate to his father's bantering approach. The question seemed to be whether Mary could cope with the strain of this. She felt that it had been a bad day because she was tired and the apprehension of how his mood would be made her more tense. We agreed that the weep in the duty room was probably a good thing, providing a safety valve. She thought that Stephen probably knew that she had been upset.

We also talked through that evening the regular bone of contention, the evening physiotherapy session. I suggested that it was important to find some way of organising the regime which would allow each of them some personal time. Donald also felt that Mary allowed Stephen to be too dependent in his personal care - "He can dress himself, he does on a Saturday". Mary admitted that she just could not stand the time it took Stephen, because he dawdled and day-dreamed, "and it's enough of a hassle getting everything done in the morning". She agreed, however, that it would pay off in the long run if she could just expect him to get dressed himself, that is, leave him to it without nagging.

I had been keeping King's conceptual frmework in mind during this interview and found it helpful in assessing the situation. The theory is based on systems thinking and the major concepts are interaction, transaction, perception, self, role, stress, growth and development, time and space*.

Stephen's self-perception was clearly important; most of the time he strove to live a normal life and refused to see himself as disabled, but when he felt really ill his perception changed. His parents' refusal to allow him to embrace the sick role led to conflict and stress, but this could be seen as constructive in terms of long-term adaptation. There was a degree of role strain for the parents, with both to an extent feeling trapped by the intense demands of the situation. This was focused on the sharing of responsibility for physiotherapy and their differing reactions to Stephen's depression. Anxiety in anticipation of loss must have been underlying the feelings of each family member, affecting communication. According to Stephen's level of growth and development his independence should have been increasing, but a combination of physical weakness, lack of motivation and pressure of time had inhibited this.

The concept of goal attainment developed in King's theory of nursing also seemed relevant and we discussed the goal of allowing independence in dressing and the value of giving Stephen a specific goal to work towards, such as an art project for the ward which would give him a challenge and help to keep him occupied. Their aim of preventing Stephen from adopting the sick role was endorsed and my aim was to reinforce their concept of themselves as good parents.

Heart-lung transplant

The initiative came from Stephen himself, early in 1988. He had been in and out of hospital every few weeks over the previous six months and, at the beginning of the week, had been trying to hold out against yet another admission. By the Wednesday he was "beyond it" and said first thing in the morning, "I'll have to go now. Liz can do my physio" (Liz was the physiotherapist who usually looked after him in hospital). He was found to have an unusual organism in his sputum which necessitated isolation; this made him very miserable. When the consultant came round Stephen said, "I want to talk to you". He went on to ask about having a heart-lung transplant. The consultant admitted to having thought about it also

---

*This section was used as the basis for a chapter in While, A. (1991) *Caring for Children Towards Partnership with Parents*. London, Edward Arnold.

and promised to get in touch with the specialist in London. "You'll need to bear with me", he said, "it'll take a long time, probably about a year".

Donald was initially not keen on the idea, but Mary said to him, "It's no us that's suffering". Mary thought that Lesley was devastated by the suggestion. She had just seen something on television about it and she said, "You're no going to let him get that done?". Mary answered, "It's Stephen's decision. After all, how would you like to live the life he's living?". She had to agree. When I said later to Mary that I thought she handled it well with Lesley, she said:

> I don't think she'd ever really stopped to think what it's like for him. She sometimes says, 'He gets all the attention', but he misses out on such a lot.

When I asked how she was herself, she said:

> I was really depressed at the weekend. I can't cope when he's greetin' all the time and hanging on. And on Thursday (when the transplant was discussed), that took the legs from me. It's such a new thing. It's fear really. People say, 'I don't know how you cope, I couldn't cope if it was my child'. But my friend said, 'Don't be silly, what do you think you'd do? Put him in a home and forget about him? You just have to cope'. And of course you do. But at the weekend I was just going about greeting, whether people were nice to me or rotten to me. When I got to work I couldn't be bothered to talk to the men. And I've never been like that before. I usually sit and have my coffee with them, and have a chat and listen to all their wee stories - after all that's what you're paid for - but I just couldn't be bothered. I went and had my coffee on my own. I thought, 'Look at him, he's 94 and still going strong'. I was so bitter. They get to know you. I went in last night and one of them said, 'Is the wee lad no well?', I just said 'Aye, he's in hospital again'.

Discussing this stage in the taped interview, Donald felt that coming to terms with the thought of transplant was as bad as being given the diagnosis of cystic fibrosis. Mary tried to explain:

> You know that he's very ill - deep down you know, but when someone actually says it to you, it's still a shock ... when (the consultant) said to me, 'You know if there was anything I could do for him I would' - that was about a week before we went south - I thought, 'Well, if he's saying that it's a hopeless case, there really can't be anything more they can do for him ...'. I thought, 'This is it, we're never going to see this operation'.

142

They did go south for assessment and came back quite excited about the prospect. Donald said that Stephen was accepting the idea of getting a new pair of lungs and that he was happy with the idea that he had a good heart to offer someone else. Anxiety had set in, however, and Donald was worried that that could "put a question mark on the transplantation". Mary said:

> I think it's only natural. I mean he desperately wants to have it done. They were very optimistic when we were down there, and explained everything that had to be done. I think it might have been me that's put all that in his mind. Because I asked, when they said they had done 22 operations and six had died, I said, 'Well, what did the six die of? What exactly happened that they died? And they said, 'Well, it was mostly technical'. So I think that though he didn't say anything at the time, that's what's been preying on his mind. When he said to me, 'When they take my heart and lungs out I'll really be dead' and I says, 'Aye, but you'll be on the life support machine', and he says, 'Aye, but what if the machine breaks down?', I think with me asking this has put all these wee doubts in his mind.

Talking with a youngster who had successfully gone through the transplant experience had been a great help to Stephen and his parents. Stephen was particularly delighted by the prospective change in body image. The girl had said, "Look, Stephen, my clubbing's gone" and displayed her now normal fingers. Mary said, "Even now, if you're talking about it, you see the grin from ear to ear, at the thought of his finger clubbing going away".

Mary had learned, however, that this girl had gone through a stage before the transplant when she just wanted to die:

> She was fed up of the whole thing. The time she was having to wait as well, it was getting her down. But she couldn't tell her Mum what was wrong wi' her, that she wanted to give up and die ... It was her Mum's friend that she told. She said she couldn't tell her Mum because she felt her Mum had been through so much, so she told her Mum's friend. But she said once she got it off her chest ... she realised she didn't want to die. She had too much to live for.

Lesley was unable to share her worry about Stephen having a transplant and it was only when she broke down in tears at school that she found a teacher she could speak to about it. Mary admitted that she had sometimes wondered, "Is she so thick that she doesn't take it in?". It was she who registered, however, that when the school teachers commented that Lesley's work, after showing initial improvement, had fallen off after Easter, the timing coincided with the trip to

London for the transplant assessment. The teacher promised to keep an eye on Lesley and asked her to come and tell her when Stephen went for the transplant. I rather regretted my remark commending the way Mary dealt with Lesley's reaction to the transplant. In retrospect, it might have been more helpful to accept Lesley's reaction and help her to talk about her feelings.

During his interview, Stephen said that he could not wait to get his transplant, but he felt that he would be worried when he had to go. He knew it would be hard work learning to breathe by himself after being on the life support machine, but he pointed out that it was already hard work when he came in to hospital fighting for breath. He had met two girls who had had transplants; one of whom was "really, really well", the other waiting for another transplant. "And your finger clubbing goes away. I'm really pleased about that. I hate it".

On one occasion I was in the ward chatting with Stephen and an older boy who had CF. It was lunch-time and Stephen had an apple on a plate. With his knife, he slashed into the apple, saying with a grin:

> See, Billy, that's what they do to you when you get a transplant. They have to divide your breast bone and open up your ribs (demonstrated on the apple).

From Billy, a comment like, "Who wants a transplant?". Stephen asked, "Would you give your heart tae somebody else?". "Yeah". "That's what I'm going to do".

While on the priority waiting list for transplant it seemed a good plan to relieve some of the anxiety of perhaps missing the vital telephone call by using a telephone page system. It was, on the whole, of great benefit but there was a false alarm on the first night of the family holiday. According to Mary, Donald's face was white while she and the children were all crying. When they discovered that it was a false alarm, the relief passed visibly over Stephen's face. Half an hour later, however, he was saying, "I wish it had been - get it over". The wait has gone on much longer than expected and the strain has continued, with Stephen spending as much time in hospital as at home. He said to Mary one day, "I dinnae ken if I'll ever get this operation".

The long wait for such a threatening event places a strain on the family which would be intolerable were it not for the hope that it offers in the face of an otherwise hopeless situation.

Hope for a cure of life-threatening illness is an essential factor in coping with the demands of daily care and the fears for the future. For the Deans, prayer for Stephen's healing was an ongoing commitment for their church group and featured strongly in their personal lives as shown before. Their minister had witnessed miraculous healing and saw this as an important part of his ministry. His invitation to Stephen to come to a healing meeting met with a refusal. Stephen contended that he had prayed for three years and nothing had happened. He felt that the way God would heal him would be through a transplant.

Mary told me that Stephen was quite upset that the minister had never mentioned the transplant when he prayed with them and that a recent conversation had resulted in a physical deterioration which was noticed by the doctor on duty. Mary said:

> Stephen prays every night - he's in a turmoil about it. I am at times too. I feel guilty about it, dunno why, because I'm believing in what Stephen's thinking and not really interested in what Adam (the minister) is trying to say. For me, if it makes him happier, that's enough for me.

My offer to have a chat with the minister about it was accepted by Mary with some relief, as she felt that she had not the knowledge to tackle him on such an issue. The minister was able to see me that day and I spoke about Stephen's illness and the effect his morale had on his physical condition. Transplant was discussed and it transpired that the minister's objection was not to transplant *per se*, but his sense that transplant could only be a temporary solution and was not the best way for Stephen. He had known of a girl with CF who had been totally restored to health by divine healing. This led in to his concern that Mary's life was absorbed in Stephen's welfare to the exclusion of all else, and that the extreme dependence which this bred was not good for Stephen. He was clearly deeply concerned for all the family's welfare and seemed open to my suggestion that his prayers might include transplant as an option which God might choose to effect Stephen's healing.

I learned at a later visit that the minister had spent two hours with Mary and they had discussed the transplant question. Still he had not prayed for it, but it seemed likely that he had arranged the visit the following day from the mother whose daughter had been healed of CF. Mary had explained Stephen's feelings to her, and she felt that if Stephen was so sure that his healing would be by transplant, that may well be right, and they prayed together accordingly.

Mary told me that the minister had raised with her the need to give Stephen up to God. She said that she knew what he meant because when there were prayers for healing she felt she should give him up, but felt that there was something else saying, "No, don't give him up", and she had not been able to. Donald then explained his feelings, that he would do all the things that needed to be done for Stephen in terms of responsibility for his care - and here there was a laughing acknowledgement that he was a bit of a pain about it - but he knew that the outcome was up to God; if it was not healing, it would still be better for Stephen. He likened it to thoughts about his own death; he knew the family would be grieving but, for him, he would hopefully be going on to something better. I picked that up, asking Mary if she had ever thought about her own death, maybe coming to terms with that had something to do with being able to hand Stephen over to God. She said she had not and we slipped into a joke about what she might decide to die of, which released the tension. Such intensely sensitive issues are extremely difficult to deal with adequately, but may be an important part of preparing for loss.

The time factor

Time impinged on the family's experience in many ways. For the parents it exerted a pressure on everyday life, from the increased "hassle" of including physiotherapy in the daily routine to the erosion of time when Stephen was in hospital. Most painful was its prognostic impact:

> I mean I know his condition is deteriorating and it's deteriorating pretty quickly, but no-one can say, 'Well, he's got three weeks or he's got three months or three years to live' - and probably that's going on in his mind as well - 'How long have I really got?'.

On a more practical level, for Stephen time in hospital was time lost from other things. Most of his hospital stays were shadowed by events he might miss if he did not get out in time - an important football match, a school choir presentation, a birthday. In the play leader's diary there was a revealing entry in April 1986:

S   I've got to be out by the 19th

PL   Your birthday?

S   Yes.

PL   You could have a party here - it could be worse.

S   What could be worse? Tell me what could be worse?

146

PL gave no answer.

S   You could be dead for your birthday. I wish my Mum would come.
     Do you think I could 'phone her?

In later years he began to enjoy school more and to work hard; consequently, time in hospital had the added drawback of causing him to lose ground in this school work. One of the major attractions of the new system of administering intravenous injections at home, particularly after he persuaded the doctors to change the timing of the injections, was that he could fit them around school times and keep up with his classmates.

Time has weighed particularly heavily since consideration of the transplant. Donald and Mary both felt that the prospect of a long and painful recovery period, and of having to be careful for so long after the operation, were factors in Stephen's anxiety. Mary had tried to encourage him:

> Even having a year of your life turned upside down is going to be worth it in the long run for what you're going to be able to do that you can't do now.

They commented that the time he would have to spend at the hospital after the transplant was also bothering him. Some months later, though, he seemed to have worked through that and was very keen to go ahead with the operation.

Basic tasks

The provision of food and shelter, nurture and affection was fully achieved, although not without difficulty. There were financial stresses and the cost of running a car, an absolute essential in Stephen's situation, was only manageable because of the Mobility Allowance. Without the contribution Mary was able to make there would have been constant difficulty; she enjoyed getting out to work but at times became quite exhausted when she was working for two or three nights a week and spending hours with Stephen in hospital.

Stephen's diet was an additional expense as he enjoyed steak or chops; nutrition was so important and his appetite so variable that Mary made every effort to buy and prepare food he would enjoy. This was perpetuated during spells in hospital, when often the family brought in food that he requested and the hospital diet was refused. Supplements were taken for a time but then rejected. Food was probably used by Stephen as a manipulative control at times, but he was genuinely keen to put on weight and to grow and ate heartily when he was feeling well.

Developmental tasks

Donald and Mary suffered deeply in their marriage with the diagnosis of CF and its genetic implications, and the loss of their baby daughter, followed so soon by the loss by each of a parent. They were able, however, to restructure their lives and ultimately to have their family. They illustrate poignantly the reality of growth through suffering and the strength that this gave them when their coping resources were again put to the test. Donald had said to Mary when she was expecting Stephen:

> We've had first-hand experience of CF, so if it's a CF child, at least we know what to expect and what to do. So it's no going to be such a big shock to us.

He felt that they were well prepared for the situation.

CF militated strongly against Stephen's growth and development, not only in the physical sense but also in his growth to independence. The physiotherapy routine required close contact between child and parent, which continued even though chest percussion was partially replaced by forced expiratory technique. It was a frequent source of conflict between husband and wife, and was a further manipulative tool for Stephen. His very frequent hospital admissions also bound him more closely to his parents, who naturally tried to be with him for a good part of each day. In view of all the invasive treatment which Stephen had to cope with in hospital, it was not surprising that he depended on them so much for support. Nevertheless, the play leader noted in July 1987 that, although he still liked to see her, there was a distancing between them - "He fluctuates between child and adult". His intelligence kept him from falling behind at school and losing touch with his friends; his humour and fun helped him to maintain good relationships with his peers.

Family functioning

The desire to found a family was paramount for Donald and Mary, and they were fully prepared to take the risks involved. When the worst happened and they were again required to face life-threatening illness in their child, they accepted their situation with courage and worked together to maintain family functioning and to provide for the growth and development of both their children. There were nevertheless times when their resources were over-stretched, as was seen in the account of the crises they encountered.

Both parents were aware of Lesley's vulnerability. Mary expressed her

148

concern that Lesley bore the brunt of the tensions the parents were experiencing. Donald had been short-tempered with her, then Mary had come home from hospital and within a minute was shouting at Lesley for "some silly wee thing - I could have cut my tongue out afterwards". There could be no doubt that she lost out in terms of parental attention but that seemed inevitable in view of the time taken up with hospital visiting. A real effort was made however to encourage her with her own interests and to share in her achievements. The fact that Lesley's school performance was so much poorer than Stephen's in spite of the time he lost did nothing for her self-confidence. As she matured, she became quite protective of her brother and looked out for him when they were both at secondary school. She learned child-rearing skills from her mother, who enjoyed looking after her niece's baby some weekends. Her guidance teacher advised her to think about child care as a future occupation.

It can be seen that the normal demands of parenting were greatly exaggerated by Stephen's illness. Communication between Stephen and his parents was open, if sometimes fraught. Lesley was less able to share her feelings. Mary felt that she and Donald were not really able to speak about their feelings together. There was certainly pressure on the marriage but the couple showed remarkable strength in the way they coped with this. Again, the fact that Donald did not react as quickly as Mary to changes in Stephen's condition, as if he hoped that by ignoring it the problem would go away, caused tension between them and reduced the support they gave to one another.

In spite of the strain they experienced, Donald and Mary maintained contact with extended family and friends, managed an occasional evening out together and joined in the life of the community where they lived.

Nursing support

It seemed to be appreciated by both parents from the beginning of our relationship that I was interested in the welfare of the whole family. We agreed to fairly regular visits on a 4-6 week basis initially; these continued for about four years. In the last period of the study, telephone calls or meetings in the ward most often replaced home visits as Mary's greatest need during the weeks that Stephen was at home was to relax and enjoy being together as a family.

In the earlier years, however, it was clear that she enjoyed being able to talk freely about Stephen, the current problems posed by his illness, her own health and the general well-being of the family. The possible prospect of adding to their family was also discussed. While she was often on her own for these visits, it was not unusual for one or both of the children to be in and, on a few occasions, Donald came home before I left. As was described above, there was a family counselling session during a particularly difficult spell when Mary felt that Donald was not giving enough time to the family. This theme recurred fairly frequently and was not fully resolved. On one occasion I suggested approaching a Marriage Guidance Counsellor - "because they prefer to see people earlier rather than later". Mary passed on my suggestion to Donald, who said, "It's not as bad as that". Mary said, "Well, I'm just telling you, I'm not having it".

The life history interview served to relieve my anxiety about their relationship. Mary chose to join in the interview with Donald, although she knew that it was focusing on his views. "You can see me any time", she said. In fact she participated in the interview too and it became a three-way conversation. The complementarity of their relationship was demonstrated quite beautifully in the way they responded to and for one another, as can be seen in some of the quotes.

On a practical level, I was able to arrange with the staff of the Out-patients' Department to supply Stephen with disposable sputum cups and to suggest the application, which was successful, for Mobility Allowance. (Mary had contact on a few occasions with the medical social worker at the hospital who was able to find some financial help). Mary was on the waiting list for pelvic repair to relieve stress incontinence. I suggested pelvic exercises which might be of some help in the meantime. She was later given an appointment with the Incontinence Adviser. There was discussion about the changes in dietary management of CF and I gave information about supplements which could be obtained on prescription. This was taken up and there was an initial improvement in weight gain, but it was not sustained as Stephen refused to take them after a while.

I had contact with Stephen's school teachers on a number of occasions; the first visit to the primary school followed a telephone call from Mary expressing concern about the supervision of meals, enzymes and physiotherapy. About a year later there was a conference to try to find a solution to Stephen's need for supervision with his physiotherapy. This situation involved a great many telephone calls to community health doctors, community nursing staff, school staff and the community physiotherapist. The solution was rather makeshift, but was the best which could be achieved in the circumstances, and involved me in a weekly visit to the school to supervise Stephen's physiotherapy. The school nurse supervised on one other day and the janitor 'looked in' on the other days. This was one occasion where I fulfilled an advocacy role for Mary in rejecting the suggestion that she should come up to the school each lunch-time to supervise Stephen's physiotherapy. I felt that this would put an unacceptable additional burden on her, apart from the way Stephen might feel about having his mother come to the school each day. The third contact was at the conference called to make arrangements for Stephen's transfer to secondary school.

There were many links with ward staff; once by telephone on Mary's behalf with a query about dilution of a drug for the nebuliser, once in person to prepare the way for Stephen's re-admission when I was aware that he was less well again at school. When a new ward sister started she asked me to fill her in on how the family was coping with the possibility of the transplant and how much Stephen knew about it. I initiated contact with the consultant on a number of occasions, to check on Stephen's progress, to hear his view on the problem about physiotherapy at school and to make the suggestion that Stephen might benefit from the Portacath implantable device, which at that time was just beginning to be used in Scotland. He was very amenable to this suggestion as there were considerable difficulties with frequent cannulation of Stephen's veins and I was able to set up a meeting with the Portacath representative. The operation was ultimately very successful. There was information-giving and discussion of this advance in treatment with nursing staff, and with Donald, who initially had reservations about it. Late in the study there was contact with the minister, who was an important source of support to the family but with whom there developed a communication problem, as has been described.

At the time of writing, Stephen is still waiting for his transplant. There was an abortive attempt which had to be abandoned at the door of the operating theatre because of misunderstanding about his maintenance drug regime. Stephen came to terms with this through the fact that, because one surgeon was on holiday, it would not have been possible to use his heart for another recipient. He said, "Well maybe next time they'll be able to use my heart for someone else".

In summary, the nursing function in relation to the families has been aimed towards facilitating the parental efforts to care for their sick child while maintaining the integrity of the family unit. Although the severity of the child's condition has varied greatly between the four families, it has been seen that the diagnosis of cystic fibrosis caused considerable stress in all cases and that nursing support had a part to play in strengthening the families' coping efforts.

Tragically, Duncan Bruce died of an overwhelming infection in 1991. He is greatly missed.

Stephen Dean has had his heart-lung transplant and is doing well.

Chapter four:
An analysis of the family experience

All cases are unique, and very similar to others.
(T. S. Eliot, The Cocktail Party)

The main objective of this study is to provide insight into the experience of families caring for a child with cystic fibrosis and their nursing support. The families' own accounts of their experience have been presented in narrative form, with minimal comment and analysis. Here the analysis is moved forward by progressive focusing, as described in Chapter 3. The characteristic 'funnel structure' has been demonstrated by the development of the research project. In the early stages, issues were identified through ongoing informal analysis of the data. These issues guided the line of enquiry by indicating the questions which needed to be asked. A further stage of analysis was required to select and order the data presented in the family profiles in a way that would illuminate and be true to each family's experience. Following lengthy reflection, a more conceptual analysis was developed and this is now presented using the framework of the research questions. Cross-case analysis is used in order to focus on each aspect of experience rather than focusing on particular families. In this way progressive focusing is demonstrated, with a gradual shift from describing events and reactions to generating concepts, and developing theoretical ideas and explanations. This includes the identification of aspects of the family experience which have particular importance for nursing, preparing the way for a deeper consideration of the nursing response.

1. How do family members respond to the genetic implications of cystic fibrosis?

> I really felt as if you were going about with two horns growing out of your head ...
> (Donald Dean)

Assault to self-image

The genetic implications came close to the dire prognosis in their painful impact on parents. Donald Dean's forthright reaction illustrates the effect on self-image and self-esteem. Human sexuality is such an integral part of self-image and involves such deep emotions that the information suggesting an inability to produce healthy children can be devastating. Prior's (1981) comment that a child affirms what is of basic importance to its parents - the femininity of the mother and the masculinity of the father - is given substance by this reaction (p.317). The personal pain as a reaction to the information about the genetic aspects of CF is compounded by the fact that family and others become aware of what is perceived as a grave defect. For many years Jan Crawford smarted under the comment, "Naebody on my side's had it", from her mother-in-law and the suspicion of infidelity. Feelings of guilt were reported but were accepted, retrospectively at least, as a normal response. The way in which the explanation was given clearly had an effect and two of the husbands referred to the way in which it was emphasised that both parents carried the defective gene, so that both were equally implicated. This helped to deflect blaming one another, with the deleterious effect this could have had on the marriage.

Frustration of generativity

A prime concern of the healthily developing adult is "... the establishing and guiding of the next generation" (Erikson, 1977, p.240). Information which strikes at that aspiration strikes at something fundamental to emotional integrity. The implications for future child-bearing were keenly felt, at least by the three couples who would have liked to increase their family size. The advice not to have any more children cut right across their natural drives and inclinations. As one father put it, "Everything was for a family". To produce a damaged child seemed much more acceptable than to have no child. The knowledge gained through prenatal diagnosis, while having the potential to provide relief from the fear of having a child with CF, can also present an agonising dilemma if the test is positive.

The implications spread wider as the siblings of the CF child reach maturity. Since identification of the CF gene, carrier testing can be offered. Identification of the carrier state in both partners may then pose the dilemma of whether or not to marry, then whether to risk pregnancy, prenatal testing and the possibility of having to decide to terminate the pregnancy. Where there is already a child with CF in the family, the decision is made more difficult by its implications; the choice of termination could be interpreted as devaluing the life of the child with CF. Awareness of this possibility could add to the burden of decision-making.

The ethical dilemmas of genetic counselling are clearly seen. Medical scientists discover information which has profound importance for the individuals concerned. It is not always reliable and it is not readily acceptable to the individual because of the dilemmas it poses in relation to important life decisions. Nevertheless, it is information which has the potential to prevent considerable suffering and, having been discovered, should surely be made available to the individuals whom it concerns. It is arguably the most sensitive of counselling areas. From each of the families there were appreciative comments on the way this aspect had been handled by medical staff, although there was not agreement all of the time with the advice given. The most helpful characteristics mentioned were the ability to listen while the couple talked through their thoughts and feelings, to provide information and to affirm the decision finally reached by the couple.

It seems important that nurses and others working on a long-term basis with families confronting the facts of genetic defect should be aware of the potential three-fold effect of such information on the individuals concerned. The assault to self-image, the frustration of generativity and the difficult decisions which have to be taken can be a source of long-term stress as well as a precipitating factor in the original crisis. Not all of the factors will be experienced by all individuals but I would suggest that they are so fundamental to the situation that they must be taken into account.

2. How do families respond to the life-threatening nature of CF?

You're frightened of what you're going to hear.
(Bill Crawford)

You just can't think about it or you couldn't get on with day-to-day life. That'd be the first way to a nervous breakdown.
(Gill Bruce)

For a parent, loss of a child is a threat to self since so much of self, physically and emotionally, is bound up in the life of a child. The situation meets Kahn and Steeves's (1986) theoretical definition of suffering as an experience in which "... some crucial aspect of one's own self, being or existence is threatened" (p.626). It is important that this suffering is recognised by health professionals so that the individual responses of parents can be recognised and psychosocial help, as well as physical care for the child, be offered.

Fear was mentioned by all the couples except the Bruces and it is significant that Gill's remark was made after the diagnosis of CF had been withdrawn. Before this time she would not have admitted fully the impact of the threat of CF. It is clear, however, that it is the life-threatening nature of the diagnosis that comprises the hazardous event, colouring the caring experience and rendering the families vulnerable to crisis. Without the grim prognosis, the burden of care would be wearying but the absence of the ultimate threat would change the nature of the experience. With the diagnosis comes the threat to emotional integrity of a parent contemplating the loss of a loved child. Even a mother with the emotional strength of Jan Crawford said in answer to a question about the worst aspect of Willie having CF, "Knowing I'm going to lose him ... I dinnae think I'll be able to cope when that happens".

The responses seen in these families are in accord with research findings discussed in Chapter 2; denial fluctuates with spells of depression and the bleak outlook is rarely mentioned. A spectrum of denial is illustrated by the families studied. The most maladaptive response is shown by the father whose refusal to accept the reality of the diagnosis threatened his son's treatment and alienated his wife. Other parents spoke of convincing themselves that the unpalatable information they had been given was somehow not quite true. Even the previous experience of losing a child did not prevent parents convincing themselves in the early years that their child had a mild case of the disease which would not have been diagnosed if their history had been unknown. The adaptive strength of denial can also be seen, reducing stress for parents by blocking out the fearsome future and allowing them to concentrate on day-to-day life and the considerable demands of care.

Fear is probably at the heart of the approach/avoidance behaviour seen in some parents and children with regard to information. While commenting that they would like more information about the illness, they choose not to explore the possible avenues for obtaining it. In this way they shield themselves from confrontation of feared issues. The three individuals, two fathers and one child with CF, who evidenced this approach were coping less effectively than others with the situation.

It is said that denial is likely to give way to depression and certainly where there is exacerbation of illness in the child, denial is no longer possible. Anxiety then runs high, with the fear that a hospital admission will be the start of the downward slide. Suicidal feelings were reported. Stress-related problems also arise in parents, for example, ulcer, back pain, fatigue and feeling 'run down'. 'Comfort eating' is not unusual, causing weight problems and potential loss of self-esteem. None of the parents in fact had been given tranquillisers or anti-depressants by their general practitioners; there seemed to be a shared acceptance, when the doctor was consulted, that they were in a difficult, worrying situation with which they were coping in an appropriate way.

Anger is a common reaction to a threatening situation and when displaced on to the spouse erupts in verbal or physical abuse. This obviously adds greatly to the stress of the situation and threatens the stability of the marriage and hence the welfare of the children. When the anger is expressed in irritation with the well siblings, it is followed by feelings of extreme guilt. Anger with medical or nursing staff was rarely expressed; only one mother did so and that was in relation to delays and conflicting information rather than a reaction to the threatening information. It is likely, however, that the more trivial cause for complaint masked the real source of tension.

Facing the facts

The comprehension by the parents of the grim prognosis does not always synchronise with the initial interview. One cannot say with certainty how much this relates to the information given, the way in which it is given or the person who gives it. What seems clear is that comprehension depends to some extent on the preparedness of the parent to hear such news, both in terms of the child's health status and the parents' defence mechanisms. Where the child appears perfectly healthy, the parents may be quite unable to accept the information and may not assimilate it until some time after the initial interview. Where there has been long-term low-level anxiety about the child's health, there is a degree of relief to have a diagnosis and treatment, mingled with the shock of the poor outlook. Jan Crawford was desperate with worry about her sick infant, fearing that he was dying, and for her a diagnosis, now matter how dire, was a profound relief. The bleak outlook was comprehended, but at that time took second place to the fact that there was treatment available. Although faced with the same facts of experience, her husband's coping repertoire prepared him less well to deal with the threat of the situation.

It may be some time before the well children fully comprehend the probable outcome of their sibling's condition. Long before that, though, they are likely to have some awareness of their parents' suffering. Their lack of understanding of the situation can be expressed in difficult behaviour, which only intensifies the difficulties the parents are experiencing. Alternatively, the anxiety can be taken inwards and the child becomes uncertain of the parents' love and lacking in self-confidence.

The difficulty which modern Western society has in dealing with the subject of death - particularly the untimely loss of a child - intensifies the pain for parents who are living in the shadow of death. The question, "Will he no' grow out o' it?", caused extreme frustration to the Deans. Denial was no longer an option for them as they watched their son's condition deteriorate and they were acutely sensitive to the reactions of others. The inability of others to face the fearful facts seemed to rub salt in the wound, although at an earlier stage in their experience Mary was hurt and shocked when a health visitor responded to the news that Stephen was ill in hospital with the comment, "Well you knew it would come to this, didn't you?". When parents' coping abilities are stretched to the limit it takes just one ill-chosen remark to upset the equilibrium.

The emotional cost of facing the facts of their experience is very considerable for these parents; where denial is possible and congruent with adaptation to the demands of treatment, it need not be discouraged. An awareness of the suffering of the parents, and its possible effect on the children, is important if nurses are to be sensitive in their approach.

3. How does time affect the way families perceive and experience the illness?

> I dread Willie's birthdays
> (Jan Crawford)

Progress and change

The passage of time is integral to the progress of the families through the stages of adaptation. With time there is a development of understanding of the reality of the situation, whether in terms of appreciating the deadly nature of the disease or of understanding that the baby will not just die in the night. In some cases it was several months before the diagnosis was accepted. The way in which the information was given intitially led some parents to put a time limit on their son's life, affecting their plans for and expectations of him; the concept of what a year might mean in the child's life was mentioned by two couples.

Essentially, the passing of time brings changes in the lives of family members and in family structure as grandparents die, children grow up, start work, marry, produce children. Time as the healer is also seen as the wounds of loss and of marred relationships are resolved. Time allows for new discoveries, raising new issues, such as the possibility of treatment for the CF male's sterility and advances in genetic research. For two families time brought a reversal of the diagnosis, changing fundamentally their view of the situation, but illustrating that one cannot go back in time and wipe out the years of anxiety or shed one's knowledge of the disease.

In childhood illness time is bound up with issues of growth and development, and the achievement of independence. That independence is compromised by the reliance on parents at least for supervision of treatment, if not for physical therapy. When the reality of illness is severe, there is profound emotional dependence on parents. The potential for conflict as the child reaches adolescence was illustrated by non-compliance with treatment. Clearly, time influenced the child's perception of his condition; two of the boys made reference to "still being able to do" something, a tacit acknowledgement that in time they may be more limited.

The growth and development of the healthy siblings is also vulnerable when there is a child with CF in the family. In the case studies two sisters were seen to experience a very stormy adolescence and unplanned pregnancy. One cannot argue a causal effect here, but it is possible that the parents' emotional turmoil and conflict, and the perceived favouritism of the child with CF, had an effect on the emotional needs and risk-taking of the siblings. There were three reports of siblings' school work suffering at some stage in the patient career. Burton (1975, p.190) pointed out that parental preoccupation of any kind is seen by children of all ages as a rejection of themselves. The reactions of some siblings in this study are congruent with that observation.

Threat and promise

Paradoxically, time offers both threat and hope. Parents perceive the passage of time as bringing the grave outcome nearer and fear of loss is nurtured by the sense of time running out. The sense that something could be happening 'for the last time' can cause deep depression. There was evidence also of the hope that time would provide a cure, helped by the awareness of changes and progress in treatment since first acquaintance with the disease. The advent of heart-lung transplant has changed the natural progress of the disease and has the potential to keep hope alive right to the end. But "hope deferred maketh the heart sick" and a child who feels desperately ill begins to despair when time goes on without the promised transplant becoming a reality.

Time is an important factor in the relationship between the family and the nurse. Understanding of the importance of time in the families' perceptions is relevant to the interaction between nurse and family. Hope is the antidote to despair and works powerfully for the child's sense of well-being. The chronicity of the illness, requiring long-term commitment between the nurse and family, raises issues of emotional involvement and of the setting and achievement of goals. These issues are further examined in Chapter 6.

4. How do family members find meaning in their experience of CF?

> God knew he'd be looked after in this family
> (Jan Crawford)

Finding meaning

Venters' (1981) study of CF families showed that an ability to endow the illness with meaning was significantly associated with a high level of family functioning, provided the explanation was owned by both parents. In this study, all of the mothers had some sense of God's will in relation to their child's illness and all mentioned prayer. Three of the families had an active church connection. Only one mother attempted a scientific explanation of the event and she carried that alongside a religious explanation. Where faith could give the certainty that even if the child died, "it'll be better for him", there was peace and enabling to deal with the demands of the present and to leave the future to God.

The fathers who could not offer any explanation for the illness situation did refer to the strength and encouragement they received by watching how their son coped with CF. Marris (1974, p.38) spoke of the importance of attachments and purposes as forming a context of meaning in life, which seems congruent with the finding that family members found strength and support from the child whose care formed an important purpose for the family.

The question of miraculous healing is little dealt with in secular literature but it is likely to be an area with a strong attraction to parents facing the threat of their child's incurable illness. While it holds out hope in such a bleak situation it can have a positive effect for the family, but when hope is disappointed, or where it is implied that if certain conditions are met healing will follow, the effect can be extremely negative. Two of the families made a move towards divine healing; in the other two families mothers prayed and believed their prayers to be answered.

159

The place of prayer

One question to be asked is why was prayer and Christian faith of importance, to a greater or lesser extent, to all of the families in an age when religious life is on the decline in Britain? Hymovich's (1985) American study showed praying to be the most frequently used coping strategy reported by parents (p.95) and Burton (1975) identified the importance of finding meaning in illness for the parents in her Northern Ireland study (p.222). These studies are not, however, set in present-day mainland Britain. It is beyond the scope of this study to examine the place of religion in British society, but the findings do give support to a growing evidence that spiritual values are still important in Western society (WHO, 1987, p.82). Since it is an area which has a direct link with the way in which families handle the knowledge of the threat to the life of their child, and to their coping abilities, it merits further thought and illumination.

Help for the helpless: purpose and privilege

Some of the biographical data in the literature review on loss indicated the importance of seeing a pattern, or a purpose, in the experience of illness. It spoke also of the importance of a sense of continuity. Part of what distinguishes human beings from animals is an ability to anticipate the future and to suffer pain in the contemplation of impending loss. For a parent considering the probable loss of a child, that suffering can be overwhelming. When a person is pushed to the limits of her endurance, she is likely to look beyond herself for strength to further endure and for light in the encircling darkness. Some of that strength may come from the spouse, family or friends, but there are depths of human need which cannot be met from purely human resources. Relief from the suffering may be found in drugs or alcohol, but the remedy is temporary and may carry along with it unwanted physical or social effects. Praying, at one level, allows one who is feeling helpless to ask for help. That was perhaps the level of relationship with God which Jan Crawford experienced, which was so much helped by the visit to Lourdes, and continued to be called upon in times of crisis. At a deeper level, it can allow the expression of thoughts and feelings to One whose understanding and love is infinite, giving the sense of relief from burden, and of self-worth and strength which Donald Dean described.

It may be that the apparent awful meaninglessness of the death of a child gives a particular impetus to the need of parents to endow the events with meaning. Their helplessness to protect their child from suffering and death is incongruent with their commitment to responsible parenthood. The emotional and cognitive dissonance resulting from this conflict requires resolution if the work of parenting is to carry on effectively. Believing that God has a purpose in allowing the

160

experience - even that they as parents are privileged to be given the care of a 'special child' - perhaps frees the paralysis of helplessness and allows them to move on with renewed strength. The difficulty in sharing with their spouse their deep fears may also be a dynamic factor in the search for a God who promises companionship in suffering.

It is not my intention to 'explain away' the spiritual experience of the parents in the study, only to examine some of the motivations which may have sensitized them to the spiritual dimension in life. It should be said also that at least one of the mothers had a life-long connection with her church, so one might expect that she would attempt to define her situation in a way which was in keeping with her established beliefs.

Since the spiritual dimension is important for some families caring for a child with CF, it seems important that nurses should have an understanding of this aspect of experience. While they may be unable to share the parent's perspective, an understanding of what it is will give a more complete picture of the family's resources.

5. What events precipitate crises in the lives of families caring for a child with CF?

The hazardous event - diagnosis

Golan's (1969) description of emotional crisis identified four components: the hazardous event; the vulnerable state; the precipitating factor; and the state of active crisis. The hazardous event which rendered all the families vulnerable, as has already been said, was the diagnosis of CF. For all the parents this was experienced as a shattering blow, although there were some feelings of relief where a diagnosis held the promise of treatment for a child who needed medical help. For just one mother, Chris Armstrong, once the gravity of the diagnosis was comprehended, there was a sense of challenge, of resolving to prove the doctors wrong by doing all she could for her son. This may have released the energies which enabled her to enjoy motherhood and encourage family activities beneficial to her son's health. She was able to say that CF had not adversely affected family life. Although the fact that ultimately Robert did not have CF has to be taken into account, for some five years the parents lived with that diagnosis, fully aware of its grave implications.

Diagnostic uncertainties in themselves caused considerable disequilibrium; it took a considerable time to assimilate and adapt to the good news of not having CF. For one family there was a year of uncertainty, swinging between relief that the diagnosis had been withdrawn and anxiety because one doctor did not agree with the reversal and a correct diagnosis remained elusive. The child was totally confused and was frequently in conflict with his mother regarding diagnosis and treatment. The loss of confidence in the medical profession was considerable and the availability of nursing support, in terms of understanding the situation and providing a link with the hospital system, was important. In such a vulnerable situation it required only a postcard changing a hospital appointment to upset the family's 'steady state'.

The protracted influence of the reactions experienced at the time of the initial crisis, and the ways in which individuals dealt with the intense feelings of disequilibrium, have been shown in the family profiles. It is very clear that intervention by a caring third party at such a time can help to facilitate an adaptive response. The importance of having someone who will listen while the painful feelings are worked through, and the value of wise intervention when there is conflict between partners, is indisputable. Such help is sometimes available to mothers from health care workers, but rarely to fathers, and more rarely still to siblings. Grandparents played a very positive supportive role in the Deans' early experience, but the availability of sympathetic extended family certainly cannot be assumed, particularly when there are genetic implications. Referral to the medical social worker often occurs only when intractable problems have occurred. The need for a family focus to nursing care for chronically ill children becomes clear.

The chronic burden of care

The crises experienced need to be seen in the context of the daily burden of care. There is the daily demand of physiotherapy sessions and, at times of illness, medical advice is sometimes to give four sessions a day. When the secretions are thick a session can take over an hour, so the investment of time and energy is very considerable. The implications for a mother who wants to take full-time work outside the home are obvious, as is the related effect on family income. The children are not invariably co-operative with regard to physiotherapy and, coupled with the potential for conflict between partners about sharing the tasks, this is one of the major sources of intra-family conflict. Supervision of enzyme replacement, vitamin supplements and diet, along with monitoring of appetite, stools and weight gain requires constant effort and militates against normalisation. Weight gain can become a preoccupation with the child also, which may be helpful but may become a source of discouragement. The constant need for care necessitates communication with school staff and arrangements to provide supervision. This was an area fraught with pitfalls, although at best it could provide considerable support to the parents.

Added to this chronic burden of care directly related to CF are the stresses of ordinary family life, of bereavements, unruly teenagers, redundancy and unemployment, health problems and temporary incapacity in the parents, anxieties about the healthy children's progress at school and the effect that family stress is having on them. Financial difficulties contributed to the cumulative burden for all the families. It is hardly surprising, when all this is taken into account, that quite minor events can cause distress of crisis proportions.

Precipitating factors - illness in the child, death of a known child, comments and reactions of peers, societal attitudes

The incidents which precipitated crises, throwing the family into disequilibrium, varied in their apparent gravity. The event appearing consistently and predictably in all four case studies was an episode of illness in the child with CF. Two parents mentioned the clutching fear - "Is this it?" - which so intensified normal parental anxiety surrounding illness of a child. An aspect of the parents' experience in relation to these episodes is the responsibility which they have to carry in relation to the ill child. There were decisions about how soon to call on medical help and occasions when parents had to assert their view against the medical opinion. When the stakes are so high such decision-making is extremely stressful. If both parents are pulling together at such times the burden is considerably eased. It is worth noting that none of the families in the study had the level of education which would have made it easy for them to challenge a medical opinion, but their knowledge of their own child and their commitment to his well-being gave them the confidence to assert parental authority.

Underlying the precipitating factor of the child's illness is again the threat to life. The more developed the resources for care of CF families become, the more those families are brought together, forming a community sharing a fearsome enemy, untimely death. The news of death of a child with CF has reverberations right round that community. A number of parents attend the funeral. For others it gives reasons to avoid contact with other CF families as much as possible, not only to protect themselves from pain but also to shield their child from confrontation with the threat to his own life. The positive aspect of this crisis event is that it can provide a learning experience for siblings or for CF children and can allow them to voice anxieties usually suppressed. Nurses working with CF families are not immune themselves to the stress of such events. While it is essential that they are aware of the probable effect on other families, on staff and children at the child's school, that they provide prompt information and offer counselling, it is also important that they have a network of support to help them to deal with their own stress.

The taunting of peers about the imminent death of the child with CF cause shock waves as parents and siblings share the distress of the affected child.

Strategies to deal with the offending children and to reassure their own child have to be worked out. Another aspect of that problem arose when the mother of a friend of the ill child wondered how to deal with his question, "Might Stephen die?". The two mothers agreed it would be better to give a negative answer, as otherwise the tendency would be to over-protect Stephen instead of enjoying a normal boyhood friendship, but that pragmatic approach may lead to difficulty later for the friend.

Finally, there were several instances where societal attitudes contributed to family stress. What has already been said about the chronic burden of care and the threat to life helps to explain the frustration and anger which parents experience when there is a lack of understanding and refusal to share responsibility for the child by teachers or leaders of organisations. Although there has been a great deal of public education about CF in recent years, parents still encounter seemingly unreasonable resistance to inclusion of the child in some activites. That resistance probably stems partly from fear, knowing the grim prognosis of CF, but having insufficient knowledge to predict risks to the particular child and therefore being unwilling to take responsibility for his welfare. Coupled with that is evidence from two of the case studies of the importance of revulsion for sputum as an irrational but significant factor in the decision-making of the person in authority. Whether this could be challenged as a basis for decision-making is uncertain, but clearly within the social context there is an educational role for the paediatric community nurse. There should be support available also to parents in their negotiations with such organisations. While it would be counter-productive for the nurse to supplant the parental role in communication with school staff, there are times when the parents' emotional involvement makes it difficult for them to argue the case for their child on objective grounds, and when they themselves require advocacy.

6. How does caring for a child with CF affect interaction patterns and the coping response of families?

What has been said about the impact of the genetic implications and the life-threatening nature of CF provides a backcloth for consideration of its effect on family interaction. The consideration of time and meaning, and the identification of crisis points also feeds in to the examination of interaction and coping in the family as a whole:

> I felt as if I'd two invalids at first.
> (Jan Crawford)

164

The precursor to change is the pre-diagnostic stage which may cause tensions because of anxiety about the child but this was not clearly shown in the case studies. The first and possibly most profound effect on family interaction occurred during the confrontational stage. What seems to be crucial for family functioning is the synchrony with which partners move through the transition from seeing themselves as a normal healthy family to accepting themselves as a family with a health problem. When the wife comes to terms with the situation before her husband there is extreme strain on the relationship, with the conflict between the parents being felt by the children. The whole family is thrown into a state of disequilibrium which may take years to resolve. Where the partners have never established a complementary communication pattern, and one prefers not to know about difficult issues in family coping, they are poorly prepared to cope with such a threat as serious illness in their child. It seems that the avoidance reaction, even though seen to be maladaptive, becomes 'set' and is repeated in the face of successive threats. It is as if the couple is locked in to an interaction pattern which bars disclosure of painful feelings.

The long-term adaptive stage with its demanding burden of care requires a high level of mutual support in the marriage partnership. In all the families the mother carried the greater part of that burden and the amount of perceived support from the husband varied. Here again synchrony between partners is important; if one partner sees deterioration and is prepared to act accordingly while the other denies the evidence and does not agree to seeking medical aid, there is conflict between the parents which is sensed by the children. Even in partnerships displaying many more strengths than weaknesses there are times when their resources are exhausted, communication is impeded and tension mounts. The intervention of a sensitive third party at such times can provide the needed catalyst to re-establish communication and free the couple to move forward together again.

Talking with children.

Communication between parents and children is frequently difficult in normal family life; when there are painful issues to be faced that difficulty is likely to be greatly exaggerated. The attempt to protect oneself and loved ones from distress leads to the "web of silence" described by Turk (1964). There was some evidence of this in the families studied, although there was also a determined effort to keep communication open, particularly on the part of the mothers. The two mothers who could share with me something of their dread of the death of their son were the two who positively encouraged their sons to talk about their fears. The two families who were less inclined to voice anxieties were the two whose children were less ill and who were subsequently found not to be suffering from CF.

There is evidence here of an intuitive response by which mothers are aware that their children are worrying silently and encourage them for their well-being to bring their anxieties into the open. While the children seem untroubled, there is a preference not to probe the sensitive areas. Most of the time it will be the task of the health care team to support the parents in their approach to the situation, but part of the value of the long-term support which nurses can offer lies in the ability to monitor the effectiveness of the chosen approach. The need for the parents to develop a flexible response which can adjust to the changes over time is also important and may require nursing intervention.

Where the parents are not in step with each other in coping with the illness situation, the effect on the family system is likely to be dire. This was shown vividly by the Crawford family, where the girls had an awareness of their parents' troubles but not a full understanding. There was sympathy for the parents mixed with confusion, blaming and anger, resentment of the loss of attention and over-protection of their brother. More adaptive responses were developed over time, but the case study emphasises the importance of including the whole family in the focus of care.

When I moan at him, he moans at the kids - so it comes back to it's my fault.
(Mary Dean)

This comment illustrates the demoralising effect of living with the constant demand and recurring stress which is the pattern of life when cystic fibrosis is worsening. "As soon as you see the sputum building up, that starts the stress again". Adaptation is virtually impossible when the stage is reached that the child is spending two weeks in and two weeks out of hospital. The development of systems which allow self-administration of intravenous antibiotics at home has alleviated this problem considerably, but the tension remains. While parents make supreme efforts to maintain normal family life and to encourage their children's social activities, the quality of family life is inevitably affected as the CF child's condition deteriorates. Figure 14 illustrates the cybernetic nature of the interaction pattern in the family system which results.

Coping responses

Among the coping responses developed by the families, denial and normalisation feature strongly together. On occasions denial was maladaptive, but it was also seen to provide strength. It facilitated the family response of tucking the knowledge out of conscious awareness and getting on with life. This could only

166

Figure 14
Impact of child's illness on family interaction: increasing stress causes a
vicious spiral of guilt and recrimination

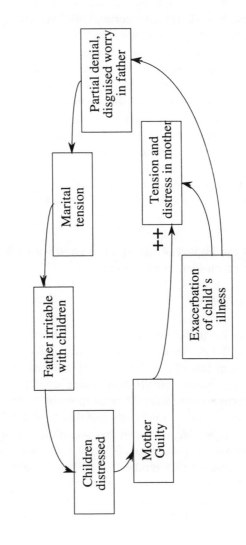

partially be effected in view of the daily burden of care as well as monthly clinic visits, but there was a clear attempt by all the families to maintain normal family life in spite of the limitations. The situation is analogous to that described by Anderson (1981, p.432) where families are in a "double bind" situation of insisting that the child is "just a normal child" yet having to impose restrictions and demands which are far from normal.

Lest the situation be presented as unrelieved gloom, it should be said that there are positive aspects to the experience of caring for a child with CF. The demands of the situation do work in some ways to bring families together. All the sisters in the study had been drawn into sharing the burden to a greater or lesser extent with their parents, some even giving the physiotherapy on occasions. In spite of the conflicts and the chronic burden, the affectional bonds remained strong in all the families and some developed tremendous strengths in coping with their situation, finding the reserves to reach beyond their own problems to the needs of others in the extended family and the wider community. The suffering is real, but so is the will to survive and to preserve the family bond.

7. What is the impact of caring for a child with CF on individual family members and on their coping response?

The affected children

This question has to include the child with CF himself, and the way he reacts to and copes with his illness. The useful role of denial has been seen whereby conscious awareness of the illness is kept to a minimum while the boys live a normal life, supporting football teams, joining in group activities and participating in such sport as they are able. They all spoke of "fighting it" and of hope for a cure. All said during the interviews that they "just didn't think about it".

On the negative side, it seemed that two of the boys had fears and anxieties, coupled with a desire to keep out of trouble, not characteristic of boys their age. There were, however, factors other than CF which could have accounted for these traits. Stephen Dean, on the contrary, was an extrovert who made up with wit, humour and well-aimed verbal attack what he lacked in energy and brawn. He battled to keep up with his peers and made friends readily, although he had to accept the painful fact that at times he was excluded from their more energetic activities. He was the one who displayed the most active coping behaviour, seeking information and attempting to control his situation, and often people within it, whether family or ward staff. He sought to understand his treatment, was prepared to question and joke with the consultant who looked after him and most of the time co-operated with the demands made on him. At times of excessive stress he could regress into less mature behaviour, letting his anger blast out at his mother and at nursing staff when he was in hospital.

The degree of autonomy which could be achieved by a 12-year old in a fairly dire situation is remarkable and is thrown into relief by comparison with Duncan Bruce, who was remarkably passive and uninvolved in the interchange during clinic visits and whose main attempt to gain control was by non-compliance with treatment. He chatted happily with clinic staff but never raised questions about his illness, although he did show an interest in technical equipment. There were, however, some signs towards the end of the study of Duncan being encouraged, to operate more independently. The severity of Stephen's condition since quite early childhood may have forced him to develop coping strategies well beyond his years, but there is clearly also the interplay between genetic endowment and the pattern of parenting which has affected the development of such different personalities and coping responses.

The mothers

The relationships which sustain the children are costly, and most particularly so for the mothers. They are first to be aware of changes in health, first to worry and to seek medical help. They undertake most of the communication with medical staff and carry the main burden of daily care. The issues discussed by Hardiker and Tod (1982) of the frustrations caused by the invisibility and the ambiguity of the illness, along with the anxieties related to its unpredictability, were illustrated in the family profiles. The employment choices for mothers are

Spells of depression are inevitable, but their commitment to the welfare of their families perhaps gives mothers the strength to maintain a positive approach in spite of their personal 'chronic sorrow'. This practical sense of purpose and the fulfilment of the mothering drive to care for and nurture children gives meaning to the situation, while the spiritual interpretation further helps to maintain coping patterns. Three of the mothers sought information through CFRT and brought it back to family members. The fact that they carried the major part of the daily burden of care also gave them a fair degree of control of the situation. All tended to put a brave face on things to the rest of the world, perhaps emphasising the threat to self-esteem which had to be counteracted by normalisation.

The fathers

The study confirms the view that fathers, too, are adversely affected by the experience of caring for a child with CF. The profoundly disturbing effects of the genetic implications and the threat to life have already been noted and, although all the fathers had reached a reasonable level of adaptation, the situation was clearly costly for them, even if they carried a relatively light proportion of the practical burden of care. A contrast can be seen here between Donald Dean, who made an effort to seek inforamtion, to draw on past experience and to maintain some mastery of the situation, and Bill Crawford, who relied largely on defence mechanisms of denial and projection, which resulted in hostility and a consequent lowering of self-esteem.

The recurring feature identified by Travis (1976, p.53) of the father abdicating responsibility and being increasingly absent from the home was only partially seen in the subject families. While work outside the home gives practical and temporal relief from the burden of care, there can be difficulties in the discontinuity of experience between the work environment and home. This is probably a phenomenon experienced by most fathers, but the tension and strain at home when there is a child with CF present a degree of role conflict far beyond the norm. Two of the fathers mentioned the difficulty of explaining to workmates what CF was and coping with their lack of understanding and interest. The heavy demand on time of home treatment and of hospital visiting was mentioned. Again, there were conflicting interests, with outside commitments to be honoured as well as household tasks which were inevitably neglected.

The siblings

The effect on siblings of distraction of parental attention to the sick child can be detrimental to their sense of self-worth and to family interaction. There is an absence of fairness in the child's view which is recurrently painful. Mixed with intensified sibling rivalry is a sharing of the parents' suffering. There are also personal anxieties in terms of how it may affect them later in life. Nevertheless, the effect seems not to be totally negative. The siblings in the study were all sisters and the development of protectiveness towards their brother may have been useful experience in preparing for motherhood.

Coping patterns often mirrored those of their parents - one might display strength and ability to share the burden with her mother, while her sister would "not get involved and bottle it up" like her father. Even the question about finding meaning brought forth a response almost identical with that of the parent they most resembled. There was deep concern for their parents also, which they found it difficult to express directly. Although all the parents tried to provide information about CF and there was family discussion about how the child was progressing, there was indeed the 'web of silence' around the threatening issues. Confrontation with the possibility of heart-lung transplant makes denial of the severity of the illness impossible to sustain and it is not surprising that Lesley Dean became depressed for a time while she was coming to terms with the new situation.

For each family member there is a personal cost in coping with the experience of CF. There are the personal implications of the genetic factor, the fears and uncertainties about the outcome, the chronic burden of care and the crisis experience; choices about work and where to live, issues of communication and disclosure. Each factor impinges on the family system as a whole, with a feedback effect on individual family members.

A major preoccupation which provided the impetus for this study was the question of nursing support for families caring for a child with CF - the needs of the families and the challenge to nursing which the situation presented. This section therefore addresses the final two research questions concerning support and points forward to the theoretical perspectives on nursing which arise from the findings.

8. What support networks do families use in relation to caring for the child with CF?

In looking at support networks one becomes aware of a range of interlinking systems, from nuclear and extended family, friends and neighbours, to groups such as Boys' Brigade, sports clubs and church fellowships, the Cystic Fibrosis Research Trust and the more formal support of the school and health care systems. Each of these systems has a life of its own, and relates to many other systems, but the interest of the study lies in examining the interchange between the family caring for the child with CF and the individuals and groups who might be expected in some way to share the burden of care. The provision of support requires first some awareness of the needs of the family, and then a willingness to look for ways to help with meeting those needs. For the sake of structuring the discussion a distinction has been made between the informal and formal network, but in reality the distinction is not clear as individuals may move across the boundaries. An example of this was a physiotherapist who had been caring for a child for some years who then stopped working but maintained contact with the family.

The informal network

Family and friends The importance of sharing the burden of care has been shown by Venters (1981), both in terms of intra-familial relationships and support from contacts outside the family. There is also evidence in the literature, however, of parents feeling isolated and unsupported (Harrisson, 1977). In examining the four case studies it can be seen that support networks changed as family structure

171

changed over time. In terms of the extended family, some grandparents had given important practical and emotional support, but some died and in one case alcoholism, remarriage and mistrust because of the genetic implications increased the vulnerability of the family. Two of the families relied to an extent on an aunt for help with child-minding.

The support of friends was appreciated but there seemed to be limits on how much practical help they could be expected to give. For one family there was a wide informal network of support, from a friend who organised her New Year party so that smokers went out to the garage and the affected child could join in the fun, to the church group who prayed and offered practical help. The parents rarely went out together, however. The difficulty of asking others to manage the physiotherapy sessions is a considerable disincentive to planning an evening out and it easily happens that couples experience a reduction in social contacts. There seems also to be a preference for being independent of outside help with practical care, which is probably an important part of the coping response, of feeling in control of the situation. For three of the families the informal network, in terms of sharing the burden of care, was restricted to the immediate family. The family boundary was relatively impermeable, although in all cases the offer of nursing support was accepted.

Neighbourhood and community Meetings of the CFRT were seen as helpful by three mothers. They provided up-to-date information and contact with other parents in a similar situation. For one mother that contact was too threatening to cope with, but her husband was actively involved.

One of the difficulties experienced in the interface between the family and the community is lack of understanding. None of the families had any previous knowledge of CF before the diagnosis, but they found public ignorance difficult to accept. The ambiguity of a chronic illness such as CF exacerbates the difficulty. The children very much want to be accepted as normal, while aware that their treatment regime and physical limitation is not normal. The unwillingness, for instance, of camp leaders to take along a child with CF illustrates the difficulty society has in coming to terms with this ambiguity. There is no doubt that those in authority can stigmatise a child with CF in a way which greatly increases the burden which the child already carries.

The formal network

The school The formal network included the health care team and the school. Communication with school staff figured in all the cases and my involvement was required in two of them. The school is a very important part of the child's life and there is potential for staff to provide valuable support or damaging disregard. A chronically ill child presents a problem to a system already stretched to cater for the needs of healthy children. The need for supervision of physiotherapy and medication poses problems when no individual can be identified to take responsibility for this. Where there is a named person who is prepared to accept responsibility for lunch-time care, a very supportive relationship can be established with both child and mother. When there was no such person available, and there was not the will in the school to make some provision, the community health team seemed unable to extend itself to meet the need fully, although the school nurse did help. Ironically, in Duncan Bruce's case the rejection in the informal network was repeated by the decision of his teacher to exclude him from the school trip abroad. This was potentially very damaging to the child's sense of self-worth, particularly occurring as it did at the threshold of adolescence. The incident caused feelings of anger, hurt and frustration for the whole family. Any expectation of support from the school system was seriously shaken.

There is an important issue here in the contradiction between a stated policy of integrating children with special needs in the general school system and the social reality when those in authority, medical advisers or teachers, are not prepared to put the policy into practice. It may be that paediatric community nurses could fulfil an advocacy role here in putting the case of a child with chronic illness so that he is allowed to participate fully in school life.

The health care team

This rather vague term requires definition. Handy's (1985) discussion of organisations equates teamwork with the task culture:

> ... the whole emphasis of the task culture is on getting the job done. To this end the culture seeks to bring together the appropriate resources, the right people at the right level of the organisation and to let them get on with it. Influence is based more on expert power than on position or personal power, although these sources have their effect. Influence is also more widely dispersed than in other cultures, and each individual tends to think he has more of it. (p.193)

This description fits neatly with the concept of a national health service and the organisation of its workforce, leaving aside the influence of political ideologies. It is perhaps less true of the organisation of nursing which tends to lean towards the role culture, with its dependence on procedures, job descriptions and authority definitions:

> Individuals are selected for satisfactory performance of a role, and the role

173

is usually so described that a range of individuals could fill it. Performance over and above the role prescription is not required, and indeed can be disruptive at times. (p.190)

The student who asks too many questions, the staff nurse who is keen to initiate change, the charge nurse who gives hours over the normal span of duty can all be seen as disruptive to the smooth running of the nursing team. Nevertheless, an appreciation of one's own role is important in multidisciplinary teamwork.

Bartlett (1961) discussed the concept of multidisciplinary teamwork from a social work perspective. She saw teamwork as a rather fluid pattern of interaction whereby two or more members of health care professions work together in the care of an individual patient. There were two basic requirements, unity of purpose and difference in knowledge and function. Each member needs to know his or her own role and competence, and each needs to understand and respect the role of others in the team:

Multidiscipline practice is a way of thinking, of keeping ideas related; a way of feeling, of readiness to share; and a way of doing, of adding one's contribution to that of others so that something larger emerges from the combination. It is a constant overweaving of all these phases of professional activity. (p.73)

When working effectively, it could well be said of the health care team that 'the whole is greater than the sum of its parts'.

(a) The medical system The medical system probably operates on the principles of Handy's (1985) task culture, although there are within it those who operate on a person culture, that is, one who does what he has to do to retain his position in the organisation but regards the organisation as:

... a base on which he can build his own career, carry out his own interests, all of which may indirectly add interest to the organisation though that would not be the point in doing them. (p.196)

The organisational structure is much looser than that of nursing, with consultants holding power and influence but doctors at registrar level having considerable influence and even junior doctors having autonomy as independent practitioners.

For the families the relationship with the hospital doctors was of supreme importance. All of the families made at least monthly visits to the clinic; there was some change over the period and some lack of continuity. Senior registrars frequently saw the child in place of the consultant and, as their posts are time-limited, some discontinuity was inevitable. One of the consultants was of the belief that since the families had to visit monthly it was important to keep the length of time to a minimum, and his sessions provided a matter-of-fact physical check-up. The pattern of such interviews was very similar to that described by Strong (1979, p.151) '... rapid, focussed and, above all, impersonal'. As Strong perceived, time belonged to the doctors rather than to the parents, and how they felt about their child, and the ups and downs of daily caring, were normally excluded.

Communication was predominantly between the mother and the doctor, but some doctors were better at including the child in the conversation than others. The most consistent and open relationship was between Stephen Dean and his consultant and increasingly as he matured Stephen spoke for himself. Medical power is an important issue raised by the case studies. It is seen at its most positive; in benign strength, giving life-long support, creating a climate in which parents and child actively participate in treatment decisions. It is also seen at its most negative; in meddlesome interference carrying out investigations with inadequate explanation, resulting in inaccurate diagnosis and unnecessary anxiety and treatment.

(b) The primary care team The aim of primary health care is to provide for the health of the community in a way which is accessible and available to all its members. The primary health care team is seen as an essential vehicle for the provision of such a community-based service (WHO, 1987). To a large extent in Britain, general practitioners, health visitors, district nurses, practice nurses and social workers share responsibility for the health of the community they serve, but communication is often lacking and the concept of teamwork can be only loosely applied (DHSS, 1986; Gilmore et al, 1974).

For three of the families the general practitioner was of much less importance than the hospital doctors in that he was seen to have a limited experience of CF and contact with the hospital was preferred. One of the families had an excellent relationship with their family doctor and trusted his word on everything related to CF, and indeed on all health matters, including emotional difficulties. None of the families had any regular contact with a health visitor, although one mother spoke warmly of the support she had received in the prediagnostic stage, which was only withdrawn because of the introduction of the home visiting nurse from the hospital.

One health visitor was contacted in relation to difficulty with supervision of physiotherapy at school, but was not keen to be involved, seeing the problem as beyond the health visiting remit. It has to be borne in mind that health visitors in this area expect there to be a specialist service from the hospital and this may serve to lessen their involvement. Nevertheless, Cull's (1974) study identified a

175

similar lack of involvement from health visitors; indeed, it was this finding which provided the stimulus for setting up a specialist home visiting nurse service. One of the children was attended by community nurses for a course of antibiotics by intramuscular injection; the drug error which occurred perhaps raises the question of the wisdom of giving nurses who do not have paediatric training the responsibility for administration of the fractional doses common in paediatric practice.

(c) The ward team The physiotherapist, the play leader and the hospital school teacher each had a unique and important role to play in the child's support network, and in some cases this developed into a friendly supportive relationship for the mother also. The physiotherapist saw the child at the clinic and, if admission was required, usually the same physiotherapist would provide most of the treatment in hospital. The closeness and continuity of this relationship was clearly a strength to children coping with the stress of illness and the discontinuity of their experience between hospital and home. The play leader was another stable figure associated with the best aspects of a hospital stay. Her creative ability and friendly interest transformed the experience for Stephen Dean and allowed the weary weeks of hospital treatment to be brightented by constructive activity and approval of his artistic abilities which increased his self-esteem. The hospital school teacher was initially resisted, but later greatly appreciated and became in a real sense a family friend in whom his mother was able to confide. There was occasional contact with a medical social worker for two of the mothers. In one case this was very much in relation to financial help; in the other, although contact seemed to be haphazard, a valuable long-term relationship existed.

The nursing team was headed by a charge nurse with specialist paediatric training, who was supported by a varying number of staff nurses, most of whom were also qualified paediatric nurses. There were usually a number of student nurses also on the ward, perhaps one nursery nurse or an enrolled nurse, and one or two nursing auxiliaries. To a large extent the nurses acted as 'gate keepers' in the ward, controlling and co-ordinating the traffic of personnel and the time schedule which shaped the children's day. They, too, set the 'atmosphere' of the ward, its child-centredness demonstrated in colourful tabards introduced - and initially made - by one charge nurse. This charge nurse and her successor were relatively stable elements in the nursing team; both showed concern and insight with regard to the family burden of CF. The acceptance of parental presence throughout a hospital stay was evident and for the child whose admissions were frequent a fair degree of privacy and personalised care was available in a side-room off the ward.

The staff nurses were a fairly mobile population but where there were frequent hospital admissions warm and supportive relationships were established. My observation of the admission procedure, involving student nurses, showed that

176

the nurses related very directly with the child and were at pains to explain the procedure and the environment. There could be some frustration however for mothers who identified areas in which the nurses were less aware of the child's reactions than they would be. To some extent this is inevitable, given the intensity of the relationship between mother and child in this context of continuous care, but it does highlight the importance of the nurse accepting the parents' expertise in the care of their own child and being prepared to refer to them when planning nursing intervention. There were instances of sensitive care, such as the nurse who spent most of the night with a child when he was moved to an unfamiliar cubicle and felt nervous and insecure. One mother commented on how much she had appreciated being offered a cup of coffee while she was sitting with her son because it indicated some human concern for her as well.

The focus of nursing care, however, was clearly the child. I was surprised on occasions to find how little awareness the ward staff nurses had of the feelings of the parents. Perhaps because the parents were mostly with their child, there seemed to be little discussion of how they themselves were coping. This was the case even in the situation in which ward staff were consistently involved in care and where there was a general sense of good and supportive relationships. Once when I was visiting Stephen Dean in hospital his mother was very weary, and told me that she had been in tears earlier, and had talked with the teacher about Stephen's irritability. The staff nurse on duty at the time knew nothing of this and asked me later if Mary did 'get uptight' about Stephen's illness as she never gave the impression that she did. I was able to explain something of the strain and anxiety that the family was undergoing at that time and felt that my contribution was accepted. There was no sense that the staff were careless of the parents' welfare, more that there was a diffidence, or a reluctance, or plain lack of opportunity to explore personal issues.

It is probably fair to comment here that for nurses, too, there are defence mechanisms which assist coping, as clearly described by Menzies (1961, p.9). While nursing has to some extent moved away from the task orientation which Menzies saw as a defence against the anxiety created by personal involvement in the suffering of patients, strategies to support and help nurses in dealing with such anxiety are only beginning to be developed in a few areas. Until there is real support for such difficulties, it is likely that defences will be used to allow avoidance of potentially distressing areas. While such defences protect the nurse from unmanageable stress, they may deny families much needed support from a source which would seem to be ideally placed to give it, since nurses are as intimately involved in the daily burden of care for the child during a spell in hospital as are the parents.

Before leaving the consideration of the support given by the health care team it is necesary to examine to what extent these health care workers did indeed function as a team. Given the principles of understanding and respect for one another's roles and of working for common goals as essential to the concept, there was evidence of a fair degree of teamwork. Consistently, however, the medical staff appeared to see themselves as leaders of the team and this was generally confirmed by the behaviour of nursing and paramedical staff, and by the view of parents. The doctor was referred to by the parents as the authority in terms of decision-making and advice, although there was an occasion when the advice of a physiotherapist was taken in preference to that of the consultant, and one mother said that she would keep her questions for a doctor or for me rather than ask nursing staff at the hospital.

My own role was somewhat ambiguous as I did not fit within the management structure and was less accessible to other members of the team than would have been the case if I had been working full-time as a paediatric community nurse. This made it difficult for some people to fit me in to the scheme of things, as evidenced by one mother asking me on several occasions, "What exactly is your job?", and a consultant thanking me courteously for taking an interest in the patient. Most of my contact with the team was initiated by me, but there were a few occasions when nursing staff or medical staff made the first approach. Mutual concern about the reactions of Duncan Bruce to the prolonged uncertainty about diagnosis after years of treatment for CF gave rise to increased communication between one of the senior registrars involved, the physiotherapist and myself; in this instance a respect for each others' roles and sharing of the goal of trying to help the family through a very difficult period was clearly evident.

There was some linking also of the school system with the health care system, in that the community paediatrician, school doctor and nurse, and community physiotherapist were all involved at one stage in discussions about the welfare and support of one of the children. My involvement in these discussions underlines the value of the kind of extension of the role of the nurse modelled by this study. While working primarily with the families and forming quite an intimate relationship with them, the nurse is able also to provide a link between the many systems which form the support network for the families.

9. What support would families caring for a child with CF like to have?

The importance of this final question is that it explores the consumers' views of the health care they experience. All of the family members had difficulty in suggesting additional measures which the health care team might provide and some indicated their satisfaction with the service offered. One affected child felt that there should be more advertising about CF so that more money would be raised for research, and that people with CF should be given a 'slip' so that if they went abroad on holiday and became sick they could have free treament! A sibling suggested more help with physiotherapy so that parents were able to go out together more easily. Another suggested a talk at the clinic for families so that they would understand more about CF and what they could do about it, "if they told them about it, it might not worry them so much". More information about research was mentioned by one father and more help with claiming benefits by a mother. A sibling felt that it would have helped if someone - "the likes of you" - had come to the school to explain about CF as she had been asked questions she felt unable to answer. "I felt guilty, thinking I'd made it sound awfy bad, and he's not bad".

The aspects of nursing support which were mentioned by the families were in relation to giving information, explaining the meaning of investigations, answering questions, listening, providing a link between the clinic and the home and between the home and the school, and providing help with child care. One mother mentioned the benefit of my involvement with CFRT activities as helping her to get involved. The ratio of all four families participating to some extent in CFRT activities is certainly not representative of the community of CF families in this area. It may be that a nurse can help parents to deal with the anxieties which CFRT meetings appear to engender sufficiently to enable them to explore the benefit from that form of support.

Information giving

Giving of information relates to answering the many questions which parents need to ask in the confrontational stage in order to fully appraise the situation and mobilise coping resources. Having opportunity to raise these questions in the relaxed environment of their own home and at their own time is felt to be beneficial. For fathers there may be no other opportunity to question health care staff and clarify their understanding of the condition. Strong's (1979) study highlighted the professionals' perception of fathers in the clinic situation, where they were generally viewed as incompetent and irrelevant (p.61). None of the fathers in this study went regularly to the clinic, although three did attend on occasions, either because the mother was unable to go or because both parents wished to be there together to receive important information. The presence of the home visiting nurse at the clinic facilitates the reinforcement of information and guards against contradictory advice. It also establishes the credibility of the nurse as part of the health care team; it was in the case where I was not regularly present at the clinic that the mother had difficulty in understanding my role.

179

Listening

The importance of listening while the many difficult areas were worked through has been evident. There is a need for a highly skilled level of counselling here so that the interaction can move from exploration of the problems to confrontation of difficult issues, the development of understanding and, where appropriate, the setting of goals. The approach used during the fieldwork was non-directive and there were few occasions when there was an explicit setting of goals. In the context of a long-term relationship this seems an appropriate strategy, but there is potential for more purposeful intervention, as will be further discussed. Since the emphasis is on including the whole family in the focus of care, an ability to work with individuals of all ages and with the family as a group is required.

Providing the link

The need for a link person working between the hospital and the home was identified by Cull (1974) and by Harris (1979) in her study of children undergoing elective surgery. The description given by Gow and Atwell (1980) of paediatric nursing in the community offers a way of meeting that need. In recent years a number of CF centres have been given financial assistance in order to establish liaison nursing posts. This study, however, highlights the complexity of the area and the importance of the nurse being equipped to help families make their way through very testing experiences in a way which protects and respects the needs of each family member and of the family unit. That being the first priority of care, it is also evident that considerable interpersonal skill is required to establish and maintain channels of communication with members of the health care team and the wider community. The personal qualities of the nurses concerned are clearly important, but they must also be helped to develop the counselling skills which will enable them to function effectively in this challenging area of care.

Helping with child care

Surprisingly, the need for help with child care, in the form of baby-sitting by someone who could give the physiotherapy to let parents go out together, was mentioned by two mothers and a sibling. While in some situations the important task may be to convince parents that they can safely leave the child in someone else's care, at times when the child's condition is deteriorating there is an understandable reluctance to pass the responsibility to friends or family. The extra needs of the child are not trivial, and the parents are aware that they have acquired nursing and physiotherapy skills in order to carry out their parental responsibilities for their sick child. These cannot readily be relinquished, leaving the child in unskilled hands. At such times the expert presence of a trained nurse would contribute greatly to the parents' peace of mind. Further, this could help to prevent social isolation and to promote healthy family functioning. Although there are initiatives within the voluntary sector to provide some support of this nature, I am unaware of involvement of qualified nurses in such a scheme. It could be difficult to co-ordinate but there is probably a need which extends to many families with a chronically ill or handicapped child. It is an organisational issue which merits further investigation.

In this chapter the data have been examined in relation to the research questions, providing an analysis of the experience of the families. An elucidation of the important area of support has been attempted and something of the consumers' perspectives on care has been portrayed. Components of nursing support have been identified and these help to provide a base for the concluding chapter in which theoretical perspectives on nursing in the context of care of chronically ill children are explained.

Chapter five:
Theory development:
Family nursing of children with chronic illness

> Begin with an assumption that whatever nursing is now ... we need to, and can, do more to improve our condition. (Styles, 1982, p.55)

Having examined the themes and issues which gave rise to the research questions, it is now appropriate to consider the contribution the study can make to the development of nursing theory. The purpose of the research was to explain and inform an area of nursing practice. It is important, therefore, to draw from the study all that serves:

> ... to orient our thinking, maybe direct further research and generally help us to conceptualise this complex business of caring. (Melia, 1982b, p.18)

Initially in this chapter the relationship of nursing practice, nursing theory and nursing research is explored. There follows an analysis of the specific areas of nursing practice described in this research, including a consideration of interpersonal relations in family nursing. The relevance of systems thinking has become increasingly clear, and provides a foundation for the theoretical perspectives elaborated. The implications of the study for nursing practice, education and management are discussed. In the concluding section the transfer of understanding from the experience of cystic fibrosis to nursing of families caring for children with other long-term health problems is considered.

The relationship of nursing practice, research and theory

The development of any field of nursing practice depends on research and theory development to provide the foundation for a body of knowledge. At an early stage in the development of nursing theory Dickoff et al (1969) commented:

> The contention here is that theory is born in practice, is refined in research, and must and can return to practice if research is to be other than a draining-off of energy from the main business of nursing and theory more than idle speculation. (p.415)

Their definition of theory was of "... an invention of concepts in interrelation" (p.419).

Batey (1977), in her review of reports in the journal *Nursing Research* was concerned about the limitations of the conceptual foundations of nursing research. She pointed out that the function of published research literature was to communicate new discoveries and insights deriving from inquiry. The objective, however, was not so much the communication as the body of knowledge itself, which was strengthened and expanded by the indentification, description and explanation of the order of the empirical world. Batey argued that the absence of conceptualisation would have an inhibiting effect on the development of theory from research (p.325). Jennings (1987) spoke of the need to interweave theory, research and practice "... as a means to increase the tensile strength of nursing science" (p.65). In an examination of successes and challenges in nursing theory development, she contended that there were encouraging areas of convergence as well as areas which did not demonstrate the strength of unification. One such area was the relationship of research and theory.

Miller (1985) was concerned about the gap between theory and practice in Britain, which she held was as great or greater than it had ever been. Severely critical of the language of much nursing theory which she believed made it inaccessible to most practising nurses, she described it as "... a beautiful fantasy which is patently unrelated to the messy, real world of nursing practice" (p.420). Miller recognised, however, that changes in health care practice had resulted in an increase in community care and greater family involvement. She conceded that:

> ... those aspects of theory which have arisen in response to changes in society will eventually have to be accommodated by changes in nursing practice, however difficult this might be for the nurse practitioners". (p.422).

Meleis (1985) provided a helpful definition of theory:

> ... a theory is an articulation and a communication of a mental image of a certain order that exists in the world, of the important components of that

order, and of the way in which those components are connected. (p.108)

She examined the tension between theorists and researchers and concluded that:

> Neither group ... has entirely completed the practice - theory - research - theory - practice cycle of developing hypotheses from theoretical propositions and refining theories by considering research results, using practice as the field from which theories evolve and for which theories are used. (p.107)

There is, however, some evidence of nurses being able to pull together in elegant research design elements of theory, research and knowledge drawn from clinical nursing. Benoliel (1977) traced her own development as a researcher and the development of studies of dying patients to illustrate the flowing kind of interaction between practice and theory which could help to explain and interpret the complex social realities of nursing, health and illness (p.112).

The present study was rooted in practice and involved observation and analysis which has generated many concepts. The progress of the study could be described as convolutionary, the term used by Meleis (1984) to identify the nature of development of the discipline of nursing. She suggested that the development of nursing has followed neither a revolutionary nor an evolutionary pattern, but rather a convolutionary process of development, representing a complex twising model rather than a linear development (p.63). She argued that it was the presence of competing theories, differing schools of thought and debatable ideas that made for scholarly activity in a discipline. While there were significant areas of agreement, that is, interest in the significance of the environment, in health and coping, in transitions and in human responses to health and illness, there had also been considerable divergence in terms of conceptual approaches and research methodologies.

I would argue that in a discipline as broad as nursing in which biological and social sciences all contribute to an understanding of the person, health, nursing and the environment - Fawcett's (1984) 'metaparadigm of nursing' - divergence of research methodologies is a strength rather than a weakness. What is important is that an appropriate strategy is chosen for the study of the particular area of interest. If the questions arise from practice, and the research yields theoretical perspectives which inform practice, nursing is strengthened in all three areas.

The development of this study has not been linear, but has moved backwards and forwards between practice and research, practice and the clarification of concepts, research and practice in a complex, winding and twisting fashion. From this process a pattern has emerged showing the interrelation of the concepts relating to family experience. The strength of systems theory as a base for family nursing has been demonstrated, firstly by explaining the 'ripple' effect of the child's illness impinging on the experience of each family member. Secondly, the input of nursing intervention to restore or maintain the equilibrium of the family system is explained.

Family nursing

The term family nursing is little used in Britain, but the concept has been inherent in the development of paediatric nursing, psychiatric nursing and health visiting over many years. Most of the thoeretical development of the concept has emanated from North America. Imogene King is one early nursing scholar whose theory has evolved to include families in the focus of care (King, 1983). Her definition of nursing is:

> ... a process of action, reaction, and interaction whereby nurse and client share information about their perceptions in the nursing situation. Through purposeful communication they identify specific goals, problems, or concerns. (King, 1981, p.2)

The emphasis on interaction relates well to the kind of nursing activity seen in this study, and in her discussion of the functions of nurses, King continues:

> Nurses are partners with physicians, with families, and the paramedical groups in the co-ordination of a plan of health care for individuals and groups. (p.9)

Travelbee's (1971) definition of nursing adds dimensions which are highly relevant:

> Nursing is an interpersonal process whereby the professional nurse practitioner assists an individual, family, or community to prevent or cope with the experience of illness and suffering and, if necessary, to find meaning in these experiences. (p.7)

This definition emphasises and links important concepts which have arisen from this study; the interpersonal nature of nursing work with families experiencing the suffering of life-threatening childhood illness, and the importance of finding meaning in that experience.

There has been increasing recognition in recent years of the significance of levels of analysis other than the individual. Family nursing literature helps to articulate this shift of focus.

> Family health is defined as a dynamic, relative state of well-being. Five dimensions - the biological, psychological, sociological, spiritual, and cultural - all combine into the holistic human system. The purpose of family nursing is to promote, maintain, and restore family health; it is concerned with the interactions between the family and society and among the family and individual family members. (Hanson, 1987, p.8)

Family health is an important concept, as the well-being of each member is influenced by the well-being of the family system as a whole. The study has shown that the health and illness of a child with cystic fibrosis profoundly influences the well-being of the parents and the siblings. The biological dimension is seen in the physical illness and the treatment regime, with the suggestion that the child's illness is at times reflected in the physical ill-health of a parent. The psychological dimension is multifaceted, encompassing the growth and development of the children, the perceptions of each family member and the dynamics of interpersonal relationships. The sociological dimension is evidenced in the availability of helpful and supportive relationships outwith the immediate family, and the interface between the family and such social systems as the school and the health care team. The importance of finding meaning in illness and prayer is evidence of the spiritual dimension. Perhaps the cultural dimension has not been explored in depth in this study but the sharing of the tasks of caring, the patterns of intra-familial interaction and the attitudes of the health care team all have a cultural basis. The five dimensions have been seen to overlap with and impinge upon one another, singly and severally affecting the family experience.

My concerns in working with the families were congruent with Hanson's (1987) statement of the purpose of family nursing, although something of Travelbee's notion of coping with the experience of illness and suffering needs to be included. Hanson commented that the goal of focusing on the family as the unit of nursing care remained an ideal more than a reality. "Family nursing as a distinct field remains in its infancy" (Hanson, 1987, p.7). Clements and Roberts (1983), however, traced the development of family nursing from the Nightingale era through public health nursing, maternal-child nursing and psychiatric nursing to its present stage of development:

> Family nursing is both innovative and conservative; it also appears rather

186

securely entrenched as one approach to nursing care in the 1980s. (p.41)

Systems thinking as a framework for family nursing

Systems theory was introduced in the literature review because of its relevance to a consideration of the family. It is clear from the family profiles and the picture that they give of the family system and its interface with wider systems that it does indeed provide a way of thinking which can help to clarify experience, and which might also serve to guide nursing intervention. Altschul (1978) suggested that for psychiatric patients a systems approach might provide a better conceptual framework for using the nursing process than one based on problem-solving or activities of daily living. The findings of this study suggest that while systems thinking does not preclude a problem-solving approach nor the use of an activities of living framework, it does offer theoretical perspectives which are particularly applicable to a supportive nursing relationship with families caring for a child with chronic illness.

It can be readily appreciated that from the early stages of interaction with the family a picture of the functioning of the family system can be drawn. The concept of wholeness is important, not just holistic care of the child who has the illness, but a holistic view of the family and the relationship of its parts. The boundaries which separate the sub-systems - child from siblings, child from parents, parents from each other - affect family interaction and are important too in separating the family system from the social system of which it remains a part. The permeability of the boundary may have profound implications for the health of family functioning. Over time it will become apparent how the family maintains homeostasis, a steady state achieved in spite of environmental stresses. Negative feedback helps to maintain stability by balancing the input and output of the system (Clements, 1983, p.64).

A relevant example is seen when a spell of illness has the effect of causing a husband to give extra attention to the sick child and to sharing the burden of care with his wife. His action has the negative feedback effect of dampening down the stress levels to more manageable proportions. The reverse happening is when the husband opts out, leaving his wife to cope unsupported with the increased demand of care, thus providing positive feedback pushing the system further away from stability.

The nurse is herself (or himself) a sub-system within the health care system. In her contact with families she may at times be drawn in, or choose to enter, the family system, affecting its homeostasis or stability. She could provide a negative feedback effect in the situation illustrated above, by compensating to some extent for the husband's deficit by providing emotional and practical support to the overburdened mother. More effectively still, she may be able to help to husband - with whom a relationship has already been established - to confront the reasons for his own behaviour and to find a more adaptive response which will contribute to family stability.

While General Systems Theory as proposed by von Bertalanffy (1966) has not attained the status of an all-explaining theory of knowledge, it has influenced the development of theoretical frameworks in a range of disciplines from business studies and information technology to sociology and nursing. Imogene King was perhaps one of the first nurses to utilise systems thinking; it was mentioned in an earlier paper in 1968 and further developed through the seventies and eighties. When, in my own practice, an activities of living model proved inadequate as a frame of reference for complex family interaction, it was King's model, with its emphasis on the interaction between personal, interpersonal and social systems, which engaged my interest and took me further in my thinking about nursing. My adaptation of the conceptual framework is illustrated in Figure 15. The central concepts of perception, self, growth and development, body image, time and space helped to extend my assessment of the child. Those of communication, role, stress, interaction and transaction gave a framework for analysis of what was going on in the family during a period of stress. Concepts of authority, power, status and decision-making were relevant to consideration of the family's interface with the school system and the medical system in particular. There were limitations, however, in that the relationship to nursing of the many concepts incorporated in the theory was not always made clear, and the emphasis on goal-attainment was not necessarily appropriate in the context of a long-term relationship with several family members.

An important contribution to this discussion is Clark's Model for Health Visiting, a British model based on systems theory (Clark, 1986). It would be reasonable for nurses reading what has been said about family nursing to conclude that this is the American parallel of health visiting in the United Kingdom. On examination of the ethos of health visiting, however, it is evident that there are important differences. Clark identified four areas in which most nursing models 'do not fit' health visiting:

1. The assumption that the focus of care is an individual person.

2. The assumption that nursing is concerned with people's problems.

3. The assumption of change.

4. The assumption of a discrete illness episode which begins at the point of admission or referral and ends at the point of discharge.

The focus on the individual and on a discrete illness episode are equally a mismatch with the nursing situation described in this study, but the concern with problems and the assumption of change are not. Clark says of the second assumption that it conflicts with the deeply held ideology of health visiting as concerned with normal healthy families who are not presenting problems (p.98). It has been clear from the data that the reason for a nurse to be involved with families caring for a chronically ill child is that they do have a serious problem with which they can be expected to need some help. On the third point Clark stated:

> The existence of a problem provides a goal for nursing intervention - to remove it, to alleviate it, or in some way to achieve change. Most of the people with whom health visitors work are healthy, and the goal of health visiting is to keep them so - in other words the goal is not change, but stability. (p.99)

While stability is a valued constituent of family life, where transitions and crises are an integral part of experience, change - indeed turbulence - is a probability and any nursing theory which can be applied to life-threatening illness must take this into account.

Brearley (1988), in a discussion of the change process, commented on the trend over time which had moved from "... relatively closed systems in a relatively stable environment towards more open systems in a much more turbulent enironment" (p.17). She suggested that changes in organisations perhaps needed to emulate the family system - "... which continuously adapts, yet holds together and has identity" (p.18). In the nursing situation which has been described, families have adapted, have held together and maintained their identity, but it is not unusual for marital breakdown to occur under such stress. Indeed the divorce rate in general, regardless of the presence of a stressor such as a chronic illness, is such that while stability may be a desired goal, helping through periods of crisis and change is, I believe, a clear requirement of nursing work with families.

As discussed in Chapter 5, the contribution of health visitors to the support of families caring for a child with cystic fibrosis has not so far been evident, and the concern more often voiced by health visitors relates to their role in health promotion than in the provision of a service for families living with chronic illness (Drennan, 1986, p.46). I would suggest therefore that it requires a professional orientation somewhat different from that of the health visitor to work with families in this situation.

Having pointed out the discrepancies between a health visiting model and the concepts underlying this nursing situation, there is much in Clark's model which

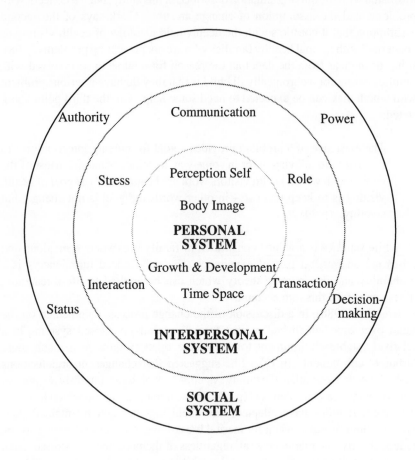

Figure 15

An adaption of King's theory of nursing as a framework for assessment

is relevant, due to its use of a systems approach and its elaboration of the interaction between the client system and the health visiting system. Clark acknowledged the contribution of King (1981) and Neuman (1982) to the development of her model. Neuman (1983) modified her systems model for work with families:

> ... the role of the nurse ... is to control vigorously factors affecting the family with special goal-directed activities toward facilitating stability within the system. (p.243)

Stability is a concept central to Neuman's work, and is considered a relative wellness state, while instability is considered an illness state. Family stressors are viewed as all forces which produce, or could produce, instability within the family system. The family as a system is classified according to psychosocial relationship characteristics, physical status, developmental characteristics and spiritual influence. Family interaction and relationship patterns are considered under the categories of individual needs, individual and composite family behavioural patterns and family adjustment needs (p.243).

Systems concepts were also applied to family interviewing by Wright and Leahey (1984). They acknowledged that the explanatory concepts of systems theory did not qualify as predictive theory, but contended that they could be used "... to explain the functioning of families and provide direction for therapeutic intervention" (p.9). The Calgary Family Assessment Model which they described, and the models presented by King, Clark and Neuman, would all be possible tools which nurses working with families caring for a sick child could use, since the basic concepts and principles are relevant to the nursing situation.

Friedemann (1989) explores the difficulty which nursing scholars have experienced in integrating the perception of family nursing practitioners, that the client is the family system rather than the individual in the family, with Fawcett's 'metaparadigm' of nursing (Fawcett, 1984). This overarching model is based on a common understanding that the concepts of person, environment, health and nursing care are the essential components of the discipline of nursing. There has been disagreement as to whether the family should be seen as the environment of the person, or as the 'person' receiving care. Friedemann argues that for the nurse to view the family simply as the environment of the person would preclude nursing intervention directed at the whole family system, while focusing on the family as the 'person' could obscure the needs of individual family members. I believe that this study supports Friedemann's view that the family must be understood as part of both concepts, of person and of environment, for a tenable theoretical base for family nursing.

The concept of family nursing is held by Friedemann to encompass three levels of the family system:

> ... nursing of the system of individuals, the system of dyads, triads and larger groups, and the entire family system. (p.212)

In individually focused family nursing the goal is personal well-being of the individuals in the family. The nurse establishes a relationship with each individual in the family and will be involved in goal setting for the health of each family member. Interpersonal family nursing encompasses the goal of mutual support and understanding among family members in addition to individual health. At this level the interpersonal family system is viewed as the client for nursing intervention which addresses family issues such as role definition and decision-making. Friedemann acknowledges the risks in this kind of nursing intervention, particularly if there is not a solid knowledge base of family and developmental theories. At the third level of family nursing practice, the client is the total system and the nursing goal is aimed at change in the system. Interventions are aimed to increase harmony between system and sub-systems as well as between system and the environment. The focus is on family health and strengths, and practice at this level requires knowledge of complex family functioning.

Friedemann's conceptualisation reflects a more advanced stage of development in thinking about family nursing than is evidenced in the British literature, but even so she accepts that ideas about family system nursing are still hazy and lacking in consensus. From the practice perspective which has emerged from this study, I would argue that the interpersonal levels and systems levels are too closely linked to be usefully differentiated.

An incident from the fourth case study serves to illustrate the point. The mother of Stephen, whose condition was deteriorating, was upset and anxious about the lack of supervision of physiotherapy at school. Stress in the mother invariably affected the other family members, particularly the spouse sub-system. It was therefore with the health of the whole family in mind that I entered into negotiations with school and community staff to work out a solution to the need for supervision of the child. The solution found was not perfect but it was sufficient to allay the mother's anxiety, providing negative feedback which helped to restore family equilibrium. This example illustrates family nursing at systems level, but includes interpersonal and individually focused care. This is congruent with Friedemann's thesis that the nurse operating at systems level will include the first two levels of practice.

The more important distinction at this stage in the development of family nursing in Britain would seem to be between viewing the child as the focus of nursing, accepting the importance of the family context, as opposed to viewing the whole family system as the unit of care. It is essential to make this distinction explicit if we are not to pay lip-service to the concept of family-focused care. This argument, however, confronts us with the centrality of interaction to the consideration of family nursing.

Interpersonal aspects of family nursing

The focus of this study is on interaction within families, between families and the social system, and between families and nurses. Miller (1985) believes that the area of nurse-patient interaction needs careful investigation by British nurse theorists. She questioned whether, in the context of British culture, values and health care system, patients wished to be active participants in care, or wished to have a close relationship with a nurse. This study supports the move towards partnership with parents which is increasingly evident in paediatric care, in that the parents undoubtedly wanted and were expected to be active participants in the management of their child's illness. It was seen, too, that a child's coping strategies could be strengthened by allowing his participation in treatment decisions. The answer to Miller's first question would seem to be that some individuals and families in Britain do indeed value a participative role in their own care, and in care of their own. Before attempting to answer Miller's second question, the kind of relationship which evolves between family and nurse requires further examination.

The human relationship

The work of those who have studied interpersonal aspects of nursing has particular relevance for family nursing. Hildegard Peplau's seminal work on interpersonal relations in nursing has recently been republished in Britain, reflecting the continuing relevance and the transcultural nature of this aspect of nursing (Peplau, 1988). In Peplau's view, the nurse-patient relationship should be educative and therapeutic:

> ... when nurse and patient can come to know and respect each other, as persons who are alike, and yet, different, as persons who share in the solution of problems. (p.9)

This statement points inescapably to a relationship between equals, and to shared decision-making, both important elements of family nursing as indicated above.

Travelbee elaborated the theme of a 'human-to-human' relationship which she held was not the same as a 'friend to friend' relationship. The differences

193

were inherent in the requirements and obligations of the participants to each other, and the element of choice in initiating and developing the relationship. She suggested that the nurse was obliged to initiate a helping process to assess needs and to seek new ways to assist. It was not essential to this process to like the recipient of care. Interpersonal closeness was likely to vary from mutual respect, to the perception of the patient or client that he or she matters to the nurse, to the possible warmth of genuine fondness (p.129).

While Miller (1985) examined the rationale for the arms-length relationship between nurses and patients which has evolved, Griffin's (1983) analysis of the concept of caring strongly challenges this approach. Griffin held that in order to be able and willing to enter into a caring relationship in which she seeks to understand the wants, desires and priorities of another, a first requirement for the nurse is what is described as "... having a good relationship with oneself". Such a relationship with oneself is a pre-requisite for sustaining a good relationship with others. Griffin then suggested that as a patient's need is perceived by the nurse, her response has several layers:

> There is the clinical assessment of what is required, the cognitive and moral recognition of the importance of the patient as a person, and significantly, the emotional element, motivating and energizing the act, and licencing us to call it caring. (p.292)

In agreement with Travelbee, Griffin believes that this emotional element does not necessarily contain the components of affection, nor of liking, although these emotions may contingently be present. The understanding of a patient's experience generates an emotion nearer to compassion. Griffin went on to identify "... the unlooked for benefits" which may accrue to a nurse. The development of a sympathetic perspective on another's feelings at a time of vulnerability, when the patient confronts the nurse with the need to act in an integrated way can put the nurse in touch with the deepest and best parts of herself - suggesting that the dominant emotion in caring is a kind of love.

In considering the nursing contribution to care, Griffin's analysis is interesting as it presents a philosopher's view of nursing and is set in the British context. I quoted it fairly substantially because it articulates values which I believe are important in nursing. Compassion for - feeling with - fellow human beings who are facing major life difficulties of illness and impending loss, and looking for ways of sustaining them in their coping efforts are fundamental to my image of nursing. While it is acknowledged that short-term contact with patients affords little opportunity for the 'enriched' kind of nursing which Griffin describes, contexts of long-term care such as care of the elderly or the chronically sick clearly do. My own experience in working with families caring for a child with cystic fibrosis has certainly been enriching and has demanded a personal commitment far beyond that which is normally expected in everyday work. Nor is this peculiar to my own experience. As one paediatric community nurse put it, "You know there's going to be a break-through. You're working so hard for them, because of the ones you've lost. You're doing it for them too".

There is evidence from the case studies and from observation of the practice of other nurses involved with families that parents appreciate having 'a knowledgeable friend' to whom they have ready access and who provides some stability in the complexities of the health care system and interlinking social systems. The answer given by this study to Miller's question about the acceptability of a close relationship between nurse and client in the British health care system is that for some families living with serious childhood illness a close relationship with a nurse forms a significant part of the family's support network.

Essentially family nursing requires a relationship of mutual respect, however far apart the nurse and the parents may be in terms of ethnic origin, educational background or social class. Both parties are committed to the welfare of the affected child but also to the well-being of the family as a whole. The situation requires "... prolonged and reliable attention" (Griffin, 1983, p.290) from parents and from nurse, probably over many years. It must be a reciprocal relationship, in which the family can consult the nurse to talk through a problem and to come to a decision, and the nurse can alert the family to a problem which she perceives.

It is not, however, a problem-driven relationship; an important part of the nurse's function is to affirm and encourage the family in its coping. It is a relationship which the nurse is required to enter to meet her professional responsibilities, regardless of her own feelings. Yet to develop and nurture the kind of relationship which will help to sustain the family through the transition from seeing themselves as a healthy family to accepting the reality of a long-term health problem and its genetic implications, through the suffering of awareness of the advancing threat of death of the child, through the crisis experiences which such families meet and to help them find meaning in it all - to do this without the energising effect of emotional involvement would not be possible. It is an experience of the fullness of life to share this journey, with the tears and laughter that are part of family life, and the hopes and the fears which are never far from the surface when such an illness is part of the matrix of family experience. It demands an emotional investment which could be called a kind of love.

If such a conclusion seems fanciful, the reader is urged to consult the paper by Menzies Lyth (1982) in which she described a piece of action research in a ward which cared for young children having long-term hospital treatment for orthopaedic problems. The project required changes in attitudes, beliefs and practices as the unit of care was consciously re-directed from the child to the family. The change in roles required a fuller deployment of the capacities of staff:

... indeed a deployment of the whole of the person in a deep, sometimes difficult, often very rewarding relationship with others ... the rewards both in increased job satisfaction and in personal growth were great. (p.37)

Such relationships have many potential tensions as is inevitable in any relationship in which human beings matter to each other. Further, wherever one who is outwith the family system seeks in some way to influence what goes on within the family, there is potential for conflict or misunderstanding.

The concept of the nurse's 'therapeutic use of self' has long been accepted in relation to psychiatric nursing, and I would suggest that it has equal importance in long-term work with families.

This analysis of caring in nursing is congruent with Fromm's (1988) theory of love as a capacity of the mature, productive character and his thesis that the art of loving can be learned by practice. Important elements in that practice were discipline, concentration and patience. A supreme concern for the mastery of any art was also seen by Fromm as a primary condition of learning, and he emphasised the life-long devotion to the art thereby required (p.92). It can be argued that mastery of the art of nursing requires just such a devotion.

Implications for nursing practice

The goal for family nursing

The nursing situation, then, is one in which nurse and parents share the goal of helping the child with CF to enjoy as healthy a life as is possible for as long as is possible. Fundamental to that goal is the maintenance of the integrity of the family unit and the well-being of each family member during that process. This assumes health - "a dynamic, relative state of wellbeing" - to be a positive value, and that the integrity of the family unit contributes to the welfare of family members. The word 'relative' is important in the context of long-term illness, and the purpose of care has to include the reality of coping with illness and its treatment and the emotional preparation for the death of the child. Although the focus of this chapter is on the nursing contribution to care, it is clear from the findings discussed in chapter 5 that many others share this goal and contribute to its realisation, for example, family, friends, school staff and other members of the health care team. In order to participate in the realisation of the goal, the nurse needs to understand and respect the contribution made by each person within the interlinking support systems. Further, she needs to be able to accept that it may be appropriate to call on another person, whether a professional or a member of the informal support network, to achieve the goals of nursing.

Nursing assessment

In family nursing it may require several visits for a full assessment of family health to be made, and initially the focus will properly be on the child who has the health problem. From the perspective of everyone in the family, that is the prime reason for the nurse's involvement. It is worthwhile, however, to make it clear at the first visit that the nurse is aware of the potential stress on the family, and is interested in the health and welfare of each family member. An Activities of Living model may be useful in making the initial assessment of the child's health and in identifying problems. The child's level of development in relation to his chronological age can also be assessed at this first visit. The model recently developed in Manchester combines activities of living and child development in its assessment stage (MacDonald, 1988). It is vitally important, however, that completing assessment schedules should not dominate the interview; establishing two-way communication which will form the basis of an open reciprocal relationship is equally important. The parent(s) and child will be making their own assessment of the nurse at this time, and it is likely to be important to them that she has expert knowledge of the child's health problem. It should be established from the beginning that the nurse is part of the health care team and provides a channel of communication to and from the family.

Parents confronting serious childhood illness are usually aware of their lack of knowledge and glad of the opportunity to air their questions. They may also need specific help with mastering new skills, or advice regarding medication or diet. Negotiation needs to take place at the end of the visit as to the purpose and frequency of visits.

Planning and implementing care

In succeeding home visits, or through contact at the clinic, the child's well-being and treatment regime is regularly checked out, but it is possible to move on to enquire about the health of the mother and to explore the family's support networks. In cystic fibrosis clinics it is usual to ensure that more than one family member is able to give physiotherapy, and it is worthwhile for the nurse to follow this up and ensure that there is indeed some sharing of the burden of care. If the husband or partner is the only other person who gives therapy, the question of further help with child care needs to be explored. If the child is of school age, it is important to find out how much communication there has been between parents and school staff, and how satisfied the parents are with the support from that area. If there is any sense of lack of understanding on the part of teaching staff, or any situation at the school which parents feel inadequate to deal with, this should be discussed and an offer of help made. It may be that the parents, having reviewed the situation, will be happy to take it further themselves, and this is to be encouraged as it confirms the parents' sense of control. If direct intervention is needed, an approach is made to school staff as the nurse provides the link between the family and the school system.

Synchrony between partners   It is particularly useful for the nurse to make early contact with each member of the family and to make it clear that she is available to answer questions or listen to problems. This is likely to require evening work but has the potential also to facilitate communication between family members, which is such an important factor in family coping. The concept of synchrony, or of 'travelling together' should be kept in mind as the nurse makes an assessment of the functioning of the family system. If it is apparent that one partner is opting out of care, or if there is obvious conflict in the marriage, it is especially important to investigate the problem sooner rather than later. It is clear that intervention at the peak of disequilibrium, that is, crisis intervention, is likely to be more effective than trying to change a maladaptive response which has become established. The intervention cannot be prescribed, but allowing each partner to express disappointment, fear, anger - and encouraging acceptance of one another's position and stage of acceptance - can help to clear the blocks in communication and understanding. A key factor is maintaining neutrality, that is, avoiding taking sides in family conflict, being "... allied with everyone and no one at the same time" (Wright and Leahey, 1984, p.103).

An illness such as cystic fibrosis raises fears and anxieties for the most mature of individuals and the most stable of marriages. Often the family nurse who has visited the home many times is the only health care professional with whom the couple has reached a level of intimacy at which it is possible to share deeply hurt feelings. It may be helpful to broach the difficult subjects of the genetic implications and the life-threatening aspects of the disease in such neutral terms as "Many parents find it really difficult to come to terms with the thought of passing an illness on to their child...". The parent will often pick up the statement and relate it to his or her own feelings. Asking the question, "What for you is the most difficult part of handling ----'s illness?", may allow the parent to put into words the dread of loss of the child.

From the data, ways in which an understanding of the situation and the family stressors involved can guide nursing intervention, have been identified. Awareness of the factors likely to precipitate crisis, for example, illness of the child, death of another child with the same condition, taunting at school, exclusion from group activity, will alert the nurse to potential problems and prompt a visit. Preparedness to move anywhere in the family's social system where an educative or advocacy role is required is important. Appreciation of the threat of the passing of time in the perception of the parents may assist sensitive interaction. The hope which

198

time can offer may be emphasised, provided it is realistic. The value of finding meaning in illness should be recognised. This cannot be forced on a family or an individual and the literature thus far provides no guidelines. Sensitive discussion of how they have managed to make sense of their situation, or find answers to the 'why?' questions may help them to think further through their suffering and find some answers which help to sustain their coping efforts. Each member of the family is likely to be helped to cope by developing some sense of control and mastery in the situation.

While the need for mothers for support in bearing their heavy share of the burden has been evidenced in this study, as in most other research in this area, the needs of fathers should not be underestimated. Perhaps they would be less inclined to opt out if they were actively included in the plan of care, sharing clinic appointments as well as the daily regime. There may be a tendency for wives to want help and yet to feel that they perform the tasks most effectively and so to exclude the husband. One father made very clear his wish to be in control of the situation and preferred to handle situations himself where his wife was happy to ask for help. The nurse needs to keep the balance of the family system in mind when offers of help are first accepted and then rejected. In this long-term relationship the nurse is likely to move in and out of the family system according to changing needs. It takes wisdom and professionalism to perceive when the family is coping well and has an effective informal support system and to decide, in consultation with the family, to reduce contact. Lines of communication need to remain open, as the stability of the situation is essentially fragile.

The well siblings The level of understanding and acceptance which the siblings have of their brother's or sister's illness should be explored. Simply alerting the parents to the likelihood of a sibling feeling rejected because of the parents' preoccupation with the sick child may be helpful, but if the situation is very fraught more specific help may be needed, otherwise such an oberservation may simply add to the parents' burden and sense of helplessness. This is an instance where mutual goal-setting can be helpful; the parent(s) and the nurse may discuss the difficulty and work out a plan whereby helathy siblings can be assured of the undivided attention of a parent on, say, two occasions each week.

The well siblings are, perhaps, the family members most vulnerable to the insecurity of lack of control, as they neither suffer the illness and its treatment directly nor carry the responsibility for care. Sharing in the treatment regimen where that is practicable is probably helpful; being prepared to call in the help of a clinical psychologist where a sibling's behaviour is causing concern over a period of months should be part of the extended role of the nurse. It is common for such referrals to require the initiative of the physician; where teamwork is fully operational this may present no problem, but it ought not to be a barrier to help for the family if the physician is not persuaded of the value of such intervention.

Evaluation: The cyclical nature of the nursing process

Evaluation can only take place when goals have been set and their achievement can be discerned. In long-term care there will not be regular setting of new goals, but the overall purpose of promoting, maintaining and restoring family health; of helping the child to enjoy as healthy a life as possible for as long as possible; of coping with the illness and the treatment regime while maintaining the integrity of the family unit and the well-being of each family member provides a standard against which the family's progress can be evaluated. The setting of short-term goals to deal with specific problems gives additional scope for evaluation of care. It is wise also to check out with the parent(s) from time to time how much contact with the nurse they feel is appropriate at the particular stage of the illness trajectory. It may well be the case that once the confrontational stage has been negotiated and the family is traversing the long-term adaptive stage, the frequency of contact can be reduced, and may indeed be maintained by telephone conversation. Regular review and consideration of the need for intervention is required, illustrating the essentially cyclical nature of the nursing process.

Within the nursing process is the principle of linking where appropriate with other members of the health care team. There is the potential for the nurse working on her own over a long period of time with families to allow the relationship to become over-dependent or, because of her familiarity with the situation, to miss a slowly developing imbalance in relationships. For these reasons, and in preparation for the possibility of no longer being available to the family for whatever reason, it would seem preferable for a second nurse to have contact with each family. Whether the nurse is based in hospital or in the community, consultation with the other health care professionals involved in the family's care is essential. This promotes consistency of information to the family and allows a sharing of knowledge within the team of carers.

The extended role of the nurse

Much has been said and written in recent years about the extended role of the nurse, but most often the extension is in terms of undertaking technical tasks which were previously the work of doctors. I would argue that there is at least as strong a case for an extension of the nurse's role in the interpersonal aspects of working with families. Feelings of uncertainty and insecurity in attempting to tackle relationship problems in families are not peculiar to nurses and should not provide the rationale for opting out. If an open and trusting relationship has been established the nurse may well be the appropriate person to offer help in the first instance. It is valuable, however, to establish links with someone experienced in marital work, for example, a social worker, clinical psychologist, family therapist or marriage counsellor. Such a person may be needed for consulation by the nurse in her supportive work with the family, and may be called in to help as co-therapist. Such links can only strengthen the support network offered by the health care team to families in trouble.

The importance of building in a support system for all staff in their work with families was emphasised by Menzies Lyth (1982, p.25); what she described as a 'talking culture' developed in the unit where the research project took place, in which important issues could be aired, confronted, and in most cases, resolved. It was seen as important that the provision for staff should match what they expected to provide for patients and families. This is a principle which badly needs to be applied in many stressful areas of nursing, but particularly in the complex area of working with families caring for a sick child.

This study highlights an important organisational issue, that is, what kind of nurse is equipped to give such care as has been described? Does the situation require a clinical specialist such as a Cystic Fibrosis Liaison Nurse, a specialist health visitor, a paediatric community nurse, or a nurse practitioner as described by Bowling and Stilwell (1988)?

As medical specialism has increased, so have nursing appointments whereby nurses provide specialist knowledge to assist patients and their relatives in the understanding and management of their condition. In the nursing situation described in this study, a Cystic Fibrosis Liaison Nurse would provide the specialist clinical knowledge necessary. A number of such appointments have been made, often funded by the CFRT, and the role was discussed by Robinson (1988). She made a very honest appraisal of the way her work had developed, admitting her own sense of inadequacy in dealing with psychological and social problems within the family. A team approach helped to resolve this difficulty, in which the nurse, a doctor, the social worker and the psychologist met to discuss particular needs and arrange appropriate intervention. Robinson maintained her view that her own training did not equip her to give the detailed psychological support some families needed, and made the point also that time spent with such families would be detrimental to work with the other families in her caseload:

> However, despite my empathy with problems such as marriages on the verge of breakdown, severely psychologically disturbed patients and relatives, financial and social upset, these all must be sorted out by the appropriate trained professional, i.e. social worker and the psychiatrist. (p.14)

This illustration of role-switching may just be acceptable in a situation where there is a specialist team to call on, but many nurses are working with children who have chronic illness, including CF, without such support. Who then will 'sort out' the problems? It is clear too from Robinson's account and from informal discussions with nurses in similar situations that the management of intravenous lines during antibiotic therapy at home is very time-consuming. In one centre it appeared that a paediatric community nurse was giving terminal care to a child with CF, while the CF liaison nurse was busy dealing with intravenous lines. Creating a specialist post, then, does not necessarily meet the requirements of the task. The holistic nature of the task needs to be fully understood, and the nurses concerned must be helped to acquire the counselling skills needed to provide family nursing.

A health visitor could be expected to have the interpersonal skills to work with the family, but there are some grounds for suspecting that few courses in health visiting provide an adequate preparation in communication with families. Certainly the input on paediatric illness does not give sufficient background knowledge to provide a resource for parents, who rapidly become knowledgeable in the field which matters so much to them. The same would be the case for the new role of nurse practitioner which may develop from the practice nurse in the United Kingdom, reflecting developments in America in the last two decades (Bowling and Stilwell, 1988).

It is evident that the individual who undertakes long-term work with families caring for a chronically ill child requires in-depth knowledge of the child's condition, of child development and family processes as well as a high level of skill in interpersonal relationships and communication. A paediatric nursing background is, I believe, an essential pre-requisite but additional preparation is necessary for the nurse to be effective at this level of interpersonal work. The extended role follows directly from the shift of focus from the ill child in his family to the family as the unit of care. This is the challenge which paediatric nursing must accept if it is to meet the needs of society and the changes in practice required by the changing patterns of care of sick children.

Transfer of understanding to other childhood illnesses

In this study systems thinking and concepts of interpersonal relations have provided a conceptual framework directly applicable to the nursing response to families dealing with cystic fibrosis. I would suggest that the study has relevance also to other life-threatening inherited childhood diseases. Cystic fibrosis has particular characteristics - a rigorous daily treatment regime, lack of visibility, the repulsiveness of sputum production, and uncertain prognosis. Other conditions such as haemophilia and muscular dystrophy have particular characteristics which must be appreciated, but there is likely to be a broadly similar effect on family functioning. Difficulty in coming to terms with genetic implications and the suffering of facing the threat of deterioration and death of a child are shared. Finding ways of adapting to the demands of care, and of coping with crises are likely to be common. Time will have a peculiar significance, and there are likely to be attempts to find meaning in the painful experience. A support network which will help in sharing the burden is likely to be important. I would suggest that the application could be made to many situations where families are confronting the problems of chronic illness.

Summary

In relation to the experience of such families it has been seen that the genetic implications of this disease can have a profound effect on the parents in terms of their self-image, and perception of their 'normal' sexuality. The frustration of generativity is a threat to emotional integrity. While genetic counselling and medical progress provide needed information and open up new possibilities, the choices which have to be made can be agonising.

The life-threatening nature of the disease causes suffering as parents face the possible loss of their child, part of themselves. Fear again threatens emotional integrity, and causes depression and maladaptive coping responses. The emotional cost of facing the facts of their experience is considerable.

Time brings changes in family structure and functioning and developmental change in the children. It allows families to work through the stages of adaptation to the illness and its implications. It contains both the threat of time running out and the hope of progress in combating the disease.

Finding meaning in illness can be a source of strength and comfort; prayer helps to counter the sense of helplessness which parents feel in being unable to protect their child from illness. There can be a sense of privilege in being trusted with the care of a child with special needs. The ill child is seen as a source of strength and support by other family members.

Families are rendered vulnerable by diagnosis of the illness, and relatively minor events precipitate crises. Frequently these incidents are of a cumulative nature, dealt with in the context of a chronic burden of daily care. Events such as an exacerbation of the illness, or the death of a known child with CF, are likely to precipitate crisis. The importance of supportive intervention at such times is evident.

A crucial factor in the way in which the family system reacts to the situation is the extent to which the family is travelling together in the stages of reaction and adaptation. If the partners are out of step with each other the effect on their relationship and on the well-being of all the children is adversely affected. A further important factor is the sense of control which parents or child feel in relation to the illness. Parental competence is evident when parents feel able to challenge medical opinion. Children are strengthened in their coping efforts when they are encouraged to participate in decision-making regarding treatment, rather than simply expected to comply.

The individual life of each family member suffers to some extent due to the illness; the affected children try not to think about their illness and set out to fight it. The siblings care deeply about the sick child but feel the effects of their parents' preoccupation with his care. Mothers carry the major part of the burden of care, and this affects their decisions about working outside the home.

Fathers share the emotional pain, although they may not be able to readily express their feelings. For them the discontinuity between work experience and home life can be difficult. There is, however, a determined effort to enjoy normal family life.

In its attempts to maintain equilibrium, the family finds support, though to a varying degree, in the social system of which it is a part. The nurse working within the health care system is a source of information, practical help and emotional support. She is available to all members of the family system and is committed to their well-being. She provides an important link between the family system and the social systems with which they interact. It is a long-term relationship requiring a high level of counselling skills and considerable emotional investment.

Conclusions and recommendations

The conclusions to which the study points relate to the need of families for support and the fitness of nursing to meet that need. There can be no doubt that the commitment of child health services in Britain to keep hospital care of children to a minimum, in recognition of the vulnerability of children to separation from family and home, results in parents carrying very considerable burdens of care for sick children. This is particularly so in chronic illness in childhood, and is made the more stressful when the illness is life-threatening. It is patently obvious that the responsibility of the health care team does not end when the child leaves hospital, but that there must be nursing support to enable parents to carry out nursing tasks. The thesis presented here is that nursing support involves a complex blend of information-giving, befriending, family counselling, and advocacy as the nurse moves in and out of the family system and links the family with support networks in the social system. The reality of the shift in focus of paediatric nursing practice from the ill child to the whole family as a unit of care must be recognised. Such recognition has considerable implications for management and education of nurses.

In earlier discussion the conclusion was reached that the appropriate nursing background for family nursing in the context of chronic illness was paediatric nursing. In their proposed reform of nursing education, the authors of the UKCC report, Project 2000 (1986), suggested that paediatric nurse education should be based on the premise that most ill children are treated at home (p.49). The intention is that the Common Foundation Programme will give a basis of understanding of "... the diverse patterns of family life" and of interpersonal communication. The Child Branch Programme will include community experience. Education of paediatric nurses in the future, then, promises to provide an appropriate preparation for work with families. I would suggest, however, that even with such a foundation, an advanced level of skill will be required to work with families in such stressful situations. It would seem to be a role for a Specialist Practitioner in Family Nursing.

The Project Group did not provide detailed guidelines for preparation of Specialist Practitioners, but they did suggest possible roles and areas of development (p.51). Health visiting was clearly seen as an area of specialism in the promotion of health and the prevention of ill-health, and specialist practitioners in district nursing, community psychiatric nursing and community mental handicap nursing were seen as necessary to give support to the new-style registered nurse practitioner. For some reason paediatric community nursing was not mentioned. It seems that, having recommended that paediatric nurses should be able to cross the boundary between hospital and community, no need for further preparation was recognised. In fairness too, the numbers of paediatric community nurses in post at the time of the discussions preparing for the Project 2000 publication were probably very small. The need for nurses with such expertise in the community is, however, increasingly being recognised.

Paediatric community nursing

Although the first paediatric community nursing services were set up and described 30 years ago, it is only recently that there has been marked growth in the number of health authorities providing such a service (Whiting, 1989). In view of the apparent 300% increase in the number of paediatric community nursing schemes in England since 1981, Whiting sought to focus attention on the educational needs of paediatric nurses working in the community. His findings show paediatric community nurses describing their activities as involvement in teaching practical procedures and general aspects of illness management, general health education, teaching fellow health professionals, wound care and administration of medications. I was concerned to note that they apparently made no mention of counselling. Since involvement in the care of children with chronic illness and of dying children was identified by almost all the community teams it is hard to believe that interpersonal work was not a part of the care given. It may be that the omission reflects the construction of the questionnaire, but it may also be that, lacking preparation in counselling skills, nurses do not recognise the importance of the listening and encouraging which they intuitively practise. It also suggests that even paediatric nurses working in the community are concentrating on the child's illness rather than the total family system. There may be an element of safety in this if nurses do not have the knowledge or skills to practice at this level, but this study has indicated something of the potential that exists for nurses to provide active support to vulnerable families.

The appointment of specialist liaison nurses for children with cystic fibrosis and other chronic conditions such as diabetes and haemophilia suggests that there is a perception that nurses are fitted for an educative and supportive role in relation to chronic illness. There is, however, as yet no appropriate education and training for this role. Paediatric nurses are required to take the District Nursing course to prepare them for community work, but this has no component for caring for sick children and their families. While it is planned to make some concession to paediatric nurses by allowing them to pursue independent child-centred study, there is no recognition of the special requirements of the work. There is an educational need here which must be met if the health service is to respond to the needs of the community it serves. The health of families is important at all levels of society, and nurses have the potential to be a valuable resource to families in difficulty due to health problems. They must be given adequate preparation to enable them to fulfil that potential.

The solution, I believe, is for the educational need to be met within the higher education sector, where a broadly based course including family studies and nursing theory, child health and illness, counselling and supervised practice would prepare a Specialised Practitioner in Family Nursing. The practitioner would work within hospital and community, being a valuable resource to hospital staff in addition to carrying a community caseload.

Suggested further research

In order to extend the body of knowledge which provides the base for practice, further research is required:

1. Replication studies looking at the experience of families caring for children with other chronic conditions such as muscular dystrophy, haemophilia and HIV infection. The ethnographic method could be used in the development of case studies. A grounded theory approach would allow comparative analysis to test some of the theoretical propositions

arising from the present study, for example, the importance of synchrony between partners for family stability. There should be a search for 'differentness' now in sampling, so that cultural differences are considered.

2.　　An action research project to develop the role of Specialist Practitioner in Family Nursing. This would involve identification of a need for nursing support for families, a review and mobilisation of resources including educational input, and a plan of action, implementation and evaluation of the plan in a cyclical process.

3.　　Phenomenological study of aspects of experience such as finding meaning in suffering. This would require in-depth interviewing with families facing life-threatening childhood illness.

The first type of study would remain close to nursing practice yet would be a rich resource for theory generation and testing. The second would facilitate an examination of nursing practice by practitioners, with the aim of enriching practice and clarifying the role of the specialist practitioner in family nursing. The third approach would help to inform a very personal and sensitive area of experience which should be understood in the context of holistic nursing.

This study has provided an analysis of a complex and specialist area of nursing. The skills required urgently require recognition and appropriate preparation of practitioners if the health service is to respond to changes in society, and within its own practice. It is not acceptable to transfer the care of ill children from hospital to home without providing effective professional support for families. On one level it is true that all nurses should practise family nursing, but in the area of chronic childhood illness expert knowledge and skills are required. Any nurse entering a long-term supportive relationship in which the family is considered the unit of care requires appropriate educational preparation and on-going emotional support. Family nursing, the logical extension of paediatric nursing, presents a challenge to nursing management, practice, research and education. It is to be hoped that, in this area, the professional potential of nursing will be actualised.

Bibliography

ALTSCHUL, A.T. (1978) A systems approach to the nursing process. *Journal of Advanced Nursing*, 3, 333-340.

ANDERSON, J.M. (1981) The social construction of illness experience: Families with a chronically ill child. *Journal of Advanced Nursing*, 6, 427-434.

ARNOLD, J.H. and GEMMA, P.B. (1983) *A child dies: A portrait of family grief*. Maryland, Aspen Systems Corporation.

BAILEY, R. and CLARKE, M. (1989) *Stress and Coping in Nursing*. London, Chapman and Hall

BARTLETT, H.M. (1961) *Social work practice in the health field*. USA, National Association of Social Workers.

BATEY, M.V. (1977) Conceptualization: Knowledge and logic guiding empirical research. *Nursing Research*, 26, 5, 324-329.

BATTEN, J.C. and MATTHEW, D.J. (1983) The respiratory system in HODSON, M.E., NORMAN, A.P. and BATTEN, J.C. (eds.) *Cystic Fibrosis*. London, Bailliere Tindall.

BECKER, H.S. (1966) cited by DENZIN, N.K. (1978) *The Research Act: A theoretical introduction to sociological methods* (2nd ed.). USA, McGraw Hill Book Co.

BECKER, H.S. (1978) The relevance of life histories in DENZIN, N.K. (ed.) *Sociological Methods: A source book*. USA, McGraw-Hill Book Co.

BENOLIEL, J.Q. (1984) Advancing nursing science: Qualitative approaches. *Western Journal of Nursing Research*, 6, 1-8.

BLACK, D. (1981) Mourning and the family in WALDROND-SKINNER, S. (ed.) *Developments in Family Therapy Theories and Applications since 1948*. London, Routledge and Kegan Paul.

BLAXTER, M. (1976) *The Meaning of Disability: A sociological study of impairment*. London, Heinemann.

BOND, S. (1978) *Processes of communication about cancer in a radiography department.* Unpublished PhD thesis, University of Edinburgh.

BOWLBY, J. (1980) *Attachment and Loss, Vol. III. Loss: sadness and depression.* Middlesex, Penguin Books.

BOWLING, A. and STILLWELL, B. (eds.) (1986) *The Nurse in Family Practice.* London, Scutari Press.

BREARLEY, J. (1988) *Attempts to understand the change process: The development of an Institute for the Caring Professions.* Paper given in Durham to the Association of Analytical Psychotherapists and Northern Association for Analytic Psychotherapy, March 1988.

BRESLAU, N., WEITZMANN, M.and MESSENGER, K. (1981) Psychologic functioning of siblings of disabled children. *Paediatrics*, 67, 3, 344-353.

BUCHANAN, M. (1977) Paediatric hospital and home care: 2. Easing the parents' problem. *Nursing Times*, Occasional Paper, March 17, 39-40.

BURTON, L. (1975) *The family life of sick children.* London, Routledge and Kegan Paul.

BYWATER, E.M. (1981) Adolescents with cystic fibrosis: Psychosocial adjustment. *Archives of Disease in Childhood*, 56, 538-543.

CAIN, A.C.and CAIN, B.S. (1964) On replacing a child. *Journal of Americal Academy of Child Psychiatry*, July, No 3, 443-456.

CAPEWELL, G. (1986) *Cystric Fibrosis.* London, Office of Health Economics.

CAPLAN, G. (1961) *An approach to community mental health.* London, Tavistock.

CLARK, J. (1986) A model for health visiting in KERSHAW, B. and SALVAGE, J. (eds.) *Models for Nursing.* Chichester, John Wiley & Sons.

CLEMENTS, I. and ROBERTS, F. (1983) *Family health - a theoretical approach to nursing care.* New York, John Wiley & Sons.

COWEN, K., MOK, J., COREY, M., MACMILLAN, H. and SIMMON, S.R. and LEVISON, H. (1986) Psychologic adjustment of the family with a member who has cystic fibrosis. *Pediatrics*, 77, 5, 745-752.

CRAFT, M. (1979) Help for the family's neglected 'other' child. *The American Journal of Maternal Child Nursing*, 4, 5, 297-300.

CRAFT, M.J., WYATT, N.and SANDELL, B. (1985) Behavior and feeling changes in siblings of hospitalized children. *Clinical Pediatrics*, 24, 7, 374-378.

CRAIG, H.M.and EDWARD, S.J.E. (1983) Adaptation in chronic illness: An eclectic model for nurses. *Journal of Advanced Nursing*, 8, 397-404.

CULL, A.M. (1974) *Study of the psychological concomitants of a chronic illness of childhood.* Unpublished PhD. thesis, University of Edinburgh.

DENZIN, N.K. (1978) *The Research Act: A theoretical introduction to sociological methods.* USA, McGraw-Hill.

DEPARTMENT OF HEALTH AND SOCIAL SECURITY (1976) *Fit for the future*. Report of the Committee on Child Health Services (The Court Report). London, HMSO.

DEPARTMENT OF HEALTH AND SOCIAL SECURITY (1986) *Neighbourhood Nursing - A Focus for Care*. Report of the Community Nursing Review (Cumberlege Report). London, HMSO.

DICKOFF, J., JAMES, P.and WIEDENBACH, E. (1968) Theory in a practice discipline: Part 1. Practice orientated theory. *Nursing Research*, 17, 5, 415-435.

DRENNAN, V. (1986) Talking with health visitors - perceptions of their work in WHILE, A. (ed.) *Research in preventive community nursing care*. Chichester, John Wiley & Sons.

DROTAR, D., DOERSHUK, C.F., STERN, R.C., BOAT, T.F., BOYER, W.and MATTHEWS, L. (1981) Psychosocial functioning in children with cystic fibrosis. *Pediatrics*, 67, 3, 338-343.

DUKES, W.F. (1965) N = 1. *Psychological Bulletin*, 64, 1, 74-79.

EISER, C. (1990) *Chronic Childhood Disease*. Cambridge University Press

ERIKSON, E.H. (1977) *Childhood and Society*. Herts, Triad/Paladin.

FARADAY, A.and PLUMMER, K. (1979) Doing life histories. *Sociological Review*, 27, 4, 773-798.

FAWCETT, J. (1984) *Analysis and evaluation of conceptual models of nursing*. Philadelphia, F A Davis Co.

FIELD, P.A., MORSE, J.M. (1985) *Nursing Research: The application of qualitative approaches*. London, Croom Helm.

FRIEDEMANN, M. (1989) The concept of family nursing. *Journal of Advanced Nursing*, 14, 211-216.

FROMM, E. (1988) *The art of loving*. London, George Allen & Unwin.

FRUDE, N. (1990) *Understanding Family Problems*. Chichester, John Wiley & Sons

GIBRON, K. (1964) *The Prophet*. London, William Heinemann Ltd.

GILMORE, M., BRUCE, N. and HUNT, M. (1974) *The work of the nursing team in general practice*. London, Council for the Education and Training of Health Visitors.

GLASER, B.G., STRAUSS, A.L. (1965) *Awareness of Dying*. Chicago, Aldine Publishing Co.

GLASER, B.G. and STRAUSS, A.L. (1967) *The discovery of grounded theory: Strategies for qualitative research*. Chicago, Aldine Publishing Co.

GLASER, B.G. and STRAUSS, A.L. (1968) *Time for Dying*. Chicago, Aldine Publishing Co.

GLADMAN, G., CONNOR, P.S., WILLIAMS, R.F. and DAVID, T.J. (1992) Controlled study of pseudomonas cepacia and pseudomonas maltophilia in cystic fibrosis. *Archives of Disease in Childhood*, 67, 192-195.

GOLAN, N. (1969) When is a client in crisis? *Social Casework,* July, 389-394.

GOLAN, N. (1978) *Treatment in crisis situations.* New York, The Free Press.

GOLAN, N. (1981) *Passing through transitions.* New York, The Free Press.

GOLD, R.L. (1958) Roles in sociological field observations. *Social Forces*, 36, 217-223.

GOW, M., ATWELL, J. (1980) The role of the children's nurse in the community. *Journal of Pediatric Surgery*, 15, 1, 26-30.

GREEN, W. (1985) *The Long Road Home.* Herts, Lion Publishing plc.

GRIFFIN, A.P. (1983) A philosophical analysis of caring in nursing. *Journal of Advanced Nursing*, 8, 289-295.

HAMILTON, V. and WARBURTON, D. (eds.) (1979) *Human Stress and Cognition.* Chichester, John Wiley & Sons.

HAMMERSLEY, M. and ATKINSON, P. (1983) *Ethnography: Principles in Practice.* London, Tavistock Publications.

HANDY, C.B. (1985) *Understanding organizations* (3rd ed.). London, Penguin Books.

HANSON, S.M.H. (1987) Family nursing and chronic illness in WRIGHT, L., LEAHEY, M. (1987) *Families and chronic illness.* Pennsylvania, Springhouse.

HARDIKER, P. and TOD, V. (1982) Social work and chronic illness. *British Journal of Social Work*, 12, 639-667.

HARRIS, A., and SUPER, M. (1987) *Cystic Fibrosis: The facts.* Oxford, Oxford University Press.

HARRIS, P. (1979) *Children, their parents and hospitals: Consumer reactions to a short stay for elective surgery.* Unpublished PhD. thesis, University of Nottingham.

HARRISSON, S. (1977) *Families in Stress: A study of the long-term medical treatment of children and parental stress.* London, Royal College of Nursing.

HILL, R. (1949) *Families under stress.* Connecticut, Greenwood Press.

HILL, S. (1974) *In the springtime of the year.* London, Hamish Hamilton.

HIROSE, T. and UEDA, R. (1990) Long-term follow-up study of cerebral palsy children and coping behaviour of parents. *Journal of Advanced Nursing* 15, 762-770

HIRSCHFELD, M.J. and KRULIK, T. (1985) Family caregiving to severely chronically ill children and the aged in KING, K. (ed.) *Recent Advances in Nursing, 13: Long-term care.* Edinburgh, Churchill Livingstone.

HYMOVICH, D.P. and BAKER, C.D. (1985) The needs, concerns and coping of parents of children with cystic fibrosis. *Family Relations*, 34, 91-97.

JENNINGS, B.M. (1987) Nursing theory development: Successes and challenges. *Journal of Advanced Nursing*, 12, 63-69.

JENNINGS, P. (1992a) Coping Mechanisms. *Paediatric Nursing*, 4, 8, 13-15.

JENNINGS, P. (1992b) Coping strategies for mothers. *Paediatric Nursing* 4, 9, 24-26.

JOHN, A.M., BRADFORD, R. (1991) Integrating family therapy into in-patient paediatric settings; a model. *Journal of Family Therapy* 13, 207-223.

KAHN, D.L. and STEEVES, R.H. (1986) The experience of suffering: Conceptual clarification and theoretical definition. *Journal of Advanced Nursing*, 11, 623-631.

KELLERMAN, J., ZELTZER, L., ELLENBERG, L., DASH, J. and RIGLER, D. (1980) Psychological effects of illness in adolescence: 1. Anxiety, self-esteem and perception of control. *Journal of Paediatrics*, 97, 1, 126-131.

KELLY, M. (1986) *Simon: Sunday's child*. Basingstoke, Marshall Morgan & Scott Publications Ltd.

KEW, S. (1975) *Handicap and family crisis*. London, Pitman.

KING, I. (1981) *A Theory for Nursing*. New York, John Wiley & Sons.

KING, I. (1983) King's Theory of Nursing in CLEMENTS, I. and ROBERTS, F. (eds.) *Family health - a theoretical approach to nursing care*. New York, John Wiley & Sons.

KING, I.M. (1968) A conceptual frame of reference for nursing. *Nursing Research*, 17, 1, 27-31.

KODAKEK, S. (1979) Family centred care of the chronically ill child. *Association of Operating Room Nurses Journal*, 30, 635-638.

KOOP, C.E., KOOP, E. (1979) *Sometimes mountains move*. Milton Keynes, Word Publishing.

KRAUSE, K. (1991) Contracting cancer and coping with it. *Cancer Nursing,* 14 (5) 240-245.

KUZEMKO, J.A, HEELEY, A.F. (1983) Diagnostic methods and screening in HODSON M E, NORMAN, A.P., BATTEN, J.C. (eds.) *Cystic Fibrosis.* London, Bailliere Tindall.

LANDAU, L.I. (1987) Cystic Fibrosis. *Medicine International*, 2, 37, 1513-1518.

LAZARUS, R.S., AVERILL, J.R., OPTON, E.M. (1974) The psychology of coping: Issues of research and assessment in COELHO, G., HAMBURG, K.D. and ADAMS, J. (eds.) *Coping and Adaptation*. New York, Basic Books.

LEBENTHAL, E. and BASELL, D. (1983) The pancreas in cystic fibrosis in LLOYD-STILL, J.D. (ed.) *Textbook of cystic fibrosis*. Bristol, John Wright.in

LEVISON, H. and TABACHNIK, E. (1983) Pulmonary physiology in HODSON, M.E., NORMAN, A.P., BATTEN, J.C. (eds.) *Cystic Fibrosis.* London, Bailliere Tindall.

LEVISON, H., TABACHNIK, E. (1983) Pulmonary physiology in HODSON, M.E., NORMAN, A. and BATTEN, J.C. (eds.) Cystic Fibrosis. London, Bailliere Tindall.

LoBIONDO-WOOD, G. and HABER, J. (1986) *Nursing Research: Critical appraisal and utilization.* St Louis, C V Mosby Co.

MCCOLLUM, A.T., GIBSON, L.E. (1970) Family adaptation to the child with cystic fibrosis. *The Journal of Paediatrics*, 77, 4, 571-578.

MCCRAE, M. (1984) Disorders of the alimentary tract in FORFAR, J.O and ARNEIL, G.C. (eds.) *Textbook of Paediatrics.* Edinburgh, Churchill Livingstone.

MCCUBBIN, M. (1984) Nursing assessment of parental coping with cystic fibrosis.*Western Journal of Nursing Research*, 6, 4, 407-418.

MACDONALD, A. (1988) A model for children's nursing. *Nursing Times*, 84, 34, 52-55.

MCHAFFIE, H. (1988) *A prospective study to identify critical factors which indicate mothers' readiness to care for their very low birthweight baby at home.* Unpublished PhD. thesis, University of Edinburgh.

MCHAFFIE, H.E. (1992) Coping - an essential element of nursing. *Journal of Advanced Nursing*, 17, p. 933-940.

MCNEMAR, Q. (1940) cited by DUKES, W.F. (1965) N = 1. *Psychological Bulletin*, 64, 1, 74-79.

MACPHAIL,W.D.(1988)*Family therapy in the community.* Oxford,Heinemann

MARRIS, P. (1974) *Loss and Change* (revised ed.). London, Routledge and Kegan Paul.

MATTSSON, A. (1972) Long-term physical illness in childhood: A challenge to psychosocial adaptation. *Pediatrics*, 50, 5.

MEIER, P., PUGH, E.J. (1986) The case study: A viable approach to clinical research. *Research in Nursing and Health*, 9, 195-202.

MELEIS, A.I. (1985) *Theoretical Nursing.* Pennsylvania, J B Lippincott Co.

MELIA, K.M. (1987) *Learning and Working: The occupational socialization of nurses.* London, Tavistock.

MELIA, K.M. (1982a) 'Tell it as it is' - qualitative methodology and nursing research: Understanding the student nurses' world. *Journal of Advanced Nursing*, 7, 327-335.

MELIA, K.M. (1982b) *A view on basic research in the science of care.* Unpublished paper given at a symposium: Basic research in the science of care. Helsinfors.

MENNIE, M., GILFILLAN, A., COMPTON, M., CURTIS, L., LISTEN, W., PULLEN, I., WHYTE D.A. and BROCK, D. (1992) Prenatal screening for cystic fibrosis. The Lancet, 340, July 25, 214-216.

MENZIES, I. (1961) *The functioning of social systems as a defence against anxiety: A report on a study of the nursing service of a general hospital.* London, Tavistock Institute of Human Relations.

MENZIES and LYTH, I. (1982) *The psychological welfare of children making long stays in hospital: An experience in the art of the possible.* Occasional Paper No 3, London, Tavistock Institute of Human Relations.

MERENESS, D.A., TAYLOR, C.M. (1978) *Essentials of psychiatric nursing* (10th ed.). St Louis, C.V. Mosby Co.

MILLER, A. (1985) The relationship between nursing theory and nursing practice. *Journal of Advanced Nursing,* 10, 417-424.

MINUCHIN, S. (1974) *Families and family therapy.* London, Tavistock.

MULLER, D.J., HARRIS, P.J., WATTLEY, L.A. (1986) *Nursing Children: Psychology, research and practice.* London, Harper & Row.

MURGATROYD, S. (1985) *Counselling and Helping.* London, Methuen, British Psychological Society.

MURPHY, L.B. (1961) Preventive implications of development in the pre school years in CAPLAN, G. (ed.) *Prevention of mental disorders in children.* New York, Basic Books.

NATIONAL COMMISSION OF CHRONIC ILLNESS (1956) cited by MAYO, L. (1956) Problem and challenge in *Guide to Action on Chronic Illness.* New York, National Health Council.

NEILL, K. (1979) Behavioral aspects of chronic physical disease. *Nursing Clinics of North America,* 14, 3, 443-456.

NEUMAN, B. (1983) Family intervention using the Betty Neuman Health-care Systems model in CLEMENTS, I.W., ROBERTS, F.B. (eds.) *Family Health: A theoretical approach to nursing care.* New York, John Wiley & Sons.

OLSHANSKY, S. (1962) Chronic sorrow: A response to having a mentally defective child. *Social Casework,* 48, 4.

OPPENHEIMER, J.R., RUCKER, R.W. (1980) The effects of parental relationships on the management of cystic fibrosis and guidelines for social work intervention. *Social Work in Health Care,* 5, 4, 409-419.

PARKES, C.M., WEISS, R.S. (1983) *Recovery from Bereavement.* New York. Basic Books Inc.

PARKES, C.M. (1971) Psycho-social transitions: A field for study. *Social Science and Medicine,* 5, 101-115.

PATTERSON, J.A. and MCCUBBIN, H.I. (1983) The impact of family life events and changes on the health of a chronically ill child. *Family Relations,* 32, 2, 255-264.

PATTON, M.Q. (1987) *How to use qualitative methods in evaluation.* California, Sage Publications.

PEARLIN, L.I., SCHOOLER, C. (1978) The structure of coping. *Journal of Health and Social Behavior*, 19, 2-21.

PEPLAU, H. (1988) *Interpersonal relations in nursing*. London, MacMillan Education Ltd.

PERLMAN, R. (ed.) (1983) Family home care: Critical issues for services and policies. *Home Health Care Services Quarterly*, 3, 3/4.

PINCUS, L. (1976) *Death and the family: The importance of mourning*. London, Faber & Faber.

POLIT, D.F. and HUNGLER, B.P. (1987) *Nursing Research: Principles and methods* (3rd ed.) Pennsylvania, J.B. Lippincott Co.

PRIOR, P.M. (1981) The death of a child. *British Journal of Social Work*, 11, 315-327.

RAEBURN, J.A. (1983) Genetics and genetic counselling in HODSON, M.E., NORMAN, A.P. and BATTEN, J.C. (eds.) *Cystic Fibrosis*. London, Bailliere Tindall.

RAPHAEL, B. (1984) *The Anatomy of Bereavement: A handbook for the caring professions*. London, Hutchinson.

ROBINSON, T. (1988) Establishing the role of a cystic fibrosis liaison nurse. *Cystic Fibrosis News*.

ROLLAND, J.S. (1988) A conceptual model of chronic and life-threatening illness and its impact on families in CHILMAN, C., NUNALLY, E.W. and COX, F.M. (eds.) *Families in Trouble Series, Vol. 2: Chronic Illness and Disability*. California, Sage Publications.

ROPER, N., LOGAN, W. and TIERNEY, A. (1980) *The Elements of Nursing*. Edinburgh Churchill Livingstone.

ROSE, M.H. (1984) The concepts of coping and vulnerability as applied to children with chronic conditions. *Issues in Comprehensive Paediatric Nursing*, 7, 177-186.

ROY, Sr. C. (1983) Roy Adaptation Model in CLEMENTS, I., ROBERTS, F. (eds.) *Family Health: A theoretical approach to nursing care*. New York, John Wiley & Sons.

SCIENCE (1989) *News and comment*. Vol. 245.

SCOTT, M. (1993) Research report: CF Gene Therapy trials approved in the USA. *CF News* Spring 1993

SEGAL, L. (ed.) (1983) *What is to be done about the Family?* Middlesex, Penguin Books.

SELIGMAN, E. (1976) *On death and survival*. London, Tavistock.

SHADY, G. (1978) Coping styles of patients with life-threatening illness: A literature review. *Essence*, 2, 3, 149-154.

SHWACHMAN, H., REDMOND, A. and KHAN, K. (1970) Studies in cystic fibrosis. *Pediatrics*, 46, 3, 335-343.

SILVERMAN, D. (1989) Telling convincing stories: A plea for cautious positivism in case studies in GLASSNER, B. and MORENO, J.D. (eds.) *The qualitative-quantitative distinction in the social sciences*. London, Kluwer Academic Publishers.

SINCLAIR, H., WHYTE, D.A. (1987) Perspectives on community care for children in BARNES, C. (ed.) *Recent Advances in Nursing*, 16. Edinburgh, Churchill Livingstone.

SINNEMA, G. (1984) The development of independence in adolescents with CF in *Proceedings of the 9th International Cystic Fibrosis Congress*, Brighton, England. Chichester, John Wiley & Sons.

SKYNNER, R. (1976) *One flesh: Separate persons*. London, Constable.

STANDING, C. (1987) The treatment of our son with CF. *Journal of the Royal Society of Medicine*, 80, Supplement No. 15, 2-4.

STEIN, R.E. and JESSOP, D.J. (1982) A noncategorical approach to chronic childhood illness. *Public Health Reports*, 97, 4, 354-362.

STEIN, R.E., JESSOP, D.J. and RIESSMAN, C.K. (1983) Health care services received by children with chronic illness. *American Journal of Diseases of Children*, 137, 225-230.

STERN, R., BOAT, T.F., DOERSHUK, C.F., TUCKER, A.S., PRIMIANO, F.P. and MATTHEWS, L.W. (1976) Course of cystic fibrosis in 95 patients, *The Journal of Pediatrics*, 89, 3, 406-411.

STRONG, P.M. (1979) *The ceremonial order of the clinic: Parents, doctors and medical bureaucracies*. London, Routledge and Kegan Paul.

STYLES, M. (1982) *On Nursing: Toward a new Endowment*. St Louis, C.V. Mosby Co.

TERKELSEN, K.G. (1980) Toward a theory of the family life cycle in CARTER, E.A. and MCGOLDRICK, M. (eds.) *The family life cycle: A framework for family therapy*. New York, Gardner Press.

THE SHORTER OXFORD ENGLISH DICTIONARY (3rd ed.) (1983) Guild Publishing.

TIZARD, J. (1978) Handicapped children: Research to improve practice in APLEY, J. (ed.) *Care of the handicapped child: A festschrift for Ronald MacKeith*. London, Heinemann, Spastics International Medical Publications.

TOWELL, D. (1975) *Understanding psychiatric nursing*. London, Royal College of Nursing.

TRAVELBEE, J. (1971) *Interpersonal aspects of nursing* (2nd ed.). Philadelphia, F A Davis Co.

TRAVELBEE, J. (1963) What do we mean by rapport? *American Journal of Nursing*, 63, 2, 70-72.

TRAVIS, G. (1976) *Chronic illness in children: Its impact on child and family*. California, Stanford University Press.

TURK, J. (1964) Impact of cystic fibrosis on family functioning. *Pediatrics*, 67- 71.

UNITED KINGDOM CENTRAL COUNCIL (1986) *Project 2000: A new preparation for practice.* London, UKCC.

UNITED KINGDOM CENTRAL COUNCIL (1993) *The Council's Proposed Standards for Post-Registration Education: Annexe three* (May)

VAN OS, D.K., CLARK, C.G., TURNER, C.W. and HERB, ST.J.J (1985) Life stress and cystic fibrosis. *Western Journal of Nursing Research*, 7, 3, 301-311.

VENTERS, M. (1981) Familial coping with chronic and severe childhood illness: The case of cystic fibrosis. *Social Science Medicine*, 15A, 289-297.

VON BERTALANFFY, L. (1968) *General Systems Theory.* New York, Brazillier.

WALTERS, S. and HODSON, M. (1987) *Fertility, pregnancy and contraception in cystic fibrosis.* Bromley, Cystic Fibrosis Research Trust.

WESTERMARCK, E. (1926) *A short history of marriage.* London, MacMillan.

WHITING, M. (1989) *Community Paediatric Nursing in England in 1988.* Unpublished MSc. thesis, University of London.

WHYTE, W.F. (1943) *Street corner society.* Chicago, University of Chicago Press.

WILL, D., WRATE, R.M. (1985) *Integrated Family Therapy: A problem-centred psychodynamic approach.* London, Tavistock.

WINNICOT, D.W. (1978) *The Piggle: An account of the psycho-analytic treatment of a little girl.* London, The Hogarth Press and the Institute of Psycho-analysis.

WORLD HEALTH ORGANISATION (1987) *People's Needs for Nursing Care: A European Study.* Copenhagen, WHO Regional Office for Europe.

WRIGHT, L. and LEAHEY, M. (1984) *Nurses and Families.* Philadelphia, F A Davis Co.

WRIGHT, L. and LEAHEY, M. (1987) *Families and Chronic Illness.* Pennsylvania, Springhouse.

YIN, R.K. (1984) *Applied Social Science Research Methods Series Vol. 5. Case study research: Design and methods.* Beverly Hills, Sage Publications.

YIN, R.K. (1981) The case study crisis: Some answers. *Administrative Science Quarterly*, 58-65.

YOUNGHUSBAND, E., BIRCHALL, D., DAVIE, R., KELLMER PRINGLE, M.L. (1970) *Living with handicap.* London, National Children's Bureau.

ZIEMER, M.M. (1982) Coping behavior: A response to stress. *Topics in Clinical Nursing*, July, 4-12.

ZORZA, R. and ZORZA, V. (1980) *A Way to Die.* London, Sphere Books Ltd.